What You Need to Know about Surrogacy, Egg Donation, and Sperm Donation

YOUR FUTURE FAMILY

The Essential Guide to Assisted Reproduction

KIM BERGMAN, PhD

Foreword by Mark Leondires, MD

PRAISE FOR
Your Future Family

"There is no better book to read about assisted reproduction. As a parent who was personally helped by Kim Bergman, I can hear her voice, her expert advice, along with her openness and honesty about the process on every page."

—Andy Cohen, Emmy Award-winning Host, Executive Producer

"*Your Future Family* contains vital information for the many couples and individuals looking to conceive a child through ART. It's filled with advice that will also help extended networks of friends, family, and community to support and collaborate with those working through this unique way of building a family."

—Rob Scheer, founder of Comfort Cases
and author of *A Forever Family*

"Kim Bergman brings cutting-edge expertise to the table with warmth, compassion, and understanding—a rare and much needed combination. *Your Future Family* makes her unique gifts of knowledge and support accessible to people everywhere. I can't recommend it highly enough."

—The Reverend Stan J. Sloan, CEO of Family Equality Council

"*Your Future Family* addresses the important, universal issues that people face when they choose to create a family with the help of others. Kim Bergman is a passionate advocate for families of all kinds, known for her honesty and integrity which shines through in these pages."

—Wendie Wilson-Miller, founder of the Society
for Ethics in Egg Donation and Surrogacy and
coauthor of *The Insider's Guide to Egg Donation*

"Kim Bergman is a passionate, honest expert in her field. The advice she offers in *Your Future Family* is both insightful and much needed in the field of reproductive medicine."

—Angela K. Lawson, PhD, Associate Professor of Obstetrics and Gynecology (Reproductive Endocrinology and Infertility), Northwestern University

"With scientific clarity and relatable personal stories, Kim Bergman brings the journey of building a family to life, clarifying what seems too complex, and bringing heart to what you fear might be entirely clinical. This book is an essential roadmap for future parents, donors, and surrogates."

—Dustin Lance Black, Oscar-winning filmmaker, and Tom Daley, world champion diver and Olympic medalist

"Kim has written an important, accessible guide filled with her brilliant insights and relatable personal stories. *Your Future Family* makes the sometimes-overwhelming topic of assisted reproduction easy to understand for anyone and everyone considering this life-affirming journey."

—Guy Ringler, MD, fertility doctor and partner at California Fertility Partners

"I had the good fortune to have Kim's help through our two surrogacy journeys. She is not only a gifted psychologist, but a true leader and pioneer in the field of assisted reproduction. This book provides you with the valuable insights she shared along the way that, until now, were only available to those lucky enough to get to work with her."

—Ryan Murphy, American screenwriter, director, and producer

"Even if you think you know everything there is to know about assisted reproduction, you should read *Your Future Family*. Dr. Bergman covers every angle—from the simplest to the most sophisticated—with candor and clarity, making this the most comprehensive guide available!"

—Richard B. Vaughn, Esq., founding partner
of International Fertility Law Group Inc.

"It can sometimes feel like you'll need a PhD in biology to navigate assisted reproduction. *Your Future Family* covers everything you need to know (and more) in a completely accessible and easy read. Kim is a resource everyone navigating this path should have in their corner."

—Scott Brown, Vice President
of Communications at California Cryobank

"An invaluable guide for all prospective parents who want to start a family through the use of assisted reproductive technology. This book addresses all aspects—emotional, scientific, legal, and financial—of this kind of journey to parenthood. For LGBTQ community members, it's an especially welcome resource."

—Glennda Testone, executive director
of NYC's LGBT Community Center

"Dr. Kim Bergman's comprehensive knowledge and experience—which she generously shares in this book—will help you navigate the intricate and challenging world of assisted reproduction. She is a trailblazer in the field but also a sensitive professional with a real understanding of basic human needs."

—Yotam Ottolenghi, chef, restauranteur, and bestselling author

YOUR FUTURE FAMILY

The Essential Guide
to Assisted Reproduction

KIM BERGMAN, PhD

Foreword by Mark Leondires, MD

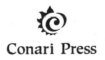

Conari Press

This edition first published in 2019 by Conari Press, an imprint of
Red Wheel/Weiser, LLC
With offices at:
65 Parker Street, Suite 7
Newburyport, MA 01950
www.redwheelweiser.com

ISBN: 978-1-57324-746-7
Library of Congress Cataloging-in-Publication Data
available upon request.

Cover design by Kathryn Sky-Peck
Cover photo by iStock/IdeaBugMedia
Interior by Steve Amarillo / Urban Design LLC
Typeset in Adobe Garamond Pro, Orpheus Pro, and Optima

Printed in Canada
MAR
10 9 8 7 6 5 4 3 2 1

*Dedicated in loving memory to Adam Gindi and
Ric Swezey and the children who call them daddy*

"A baby will make love stronger, days shorter, nights longer, bankroll smaller, home happier, clothes shabbier, the past forgotten, and the future worth living."

— Anonymous

Contents

Foreword

ONCE UPON A TIME, egg donation, sperm donation, and surrogacy were the stuff of science fiction. It was something that might happen in the far-off future when medical technology and societal mores evolved in ways that turned *The Handmaid's Tale* from novel to necessity. Fortunately, that dystopian world has not come to pass. Medical obstacles have been removed one by one, and today anyone who wants to be a parent can become one. Regardless of your sex, whether you are partnered or single, gay or straight, sexually active or asexual, becoming a parent is achievable.

Reproductive science has given us the ability to retrieve sperm and eggs, and to assess, fertilize, and successfully transfer an embryo. Surrogacy has changed the landscape of options for parents to be and has helped tens of thousands of people become parents. Assisted reproduction has changed the way we build our families, and as medical technology evolves, the odds of success will continue to improve.

That said, there are no guarantees, and there are many twists and turns on this path to parenthood. There are important questions you should ponder early on, and of course there are financial and legal considerations. But for those people who could not otherwise conceive, carry, or give birth to a child, the chance itself is incredible.

Before you embark on this journey, should you decide that it is the right path for you, it is imperative that you familiarize yourself with all aspects of the process—from the types of doctors you'll be working with and the options you have to the challenges you'll face and the laws that might affect you and the family you are committing to building. To this end, Dr. Kim Bergman has written this book.

Kim is an expert on the historically groundbreaking topic of parenting by choice, especially within the LGBTQ and infertile communities. She knows the medical science, she understands the complexity of the laws, and her wise counsel helps people handle the unique situations that assisted reproduction presents. She is an acknowledged leader in the field, regularly writing, researching, teaching, and speaking about ethical family building in the United States and abroad.

I can't think of anyone better qualified than Kim to write this book, and I am delighted that she has done so. The information is accurate, sorely needed, and highly useful to anyone and everyone interested in building a family through assisted reproduction. Kim's unwavering commitment to helping people navigate what can be an uncertain and stressful process shines through in these pages. And her open and honest approach to the topic is just what the doctor ordered.

Mark Leondires, MD

Reproductive Medicine Associates of Connecticut

Incoming Chair, LGBTQ Special Interest Group, ASRM

Founder, Gay Parents To Be

Introduction

IF YOU PICKED up this book, chances are good that you are thinking about building a family. You've been dreaming about your baby, first smiles and first steps, family vacations and holidays spent together. As with any dream, you might need some help to fulfill it. Thanks to advancements in medical technology, assisted reproductive technologies (ART) can help make your dream a reality. In these pages, I will walk you through the essential aspects of assisted reproduction, review your options, and offer you guidance on what can seem like a daunting, complicated, and mysterious process. In addition to legal and financial considerations, there are psychological issues that must be handled with care. But while the journey is complex, with thoughtful planning, it is entirely doable.

In the chapters that follow I'll outline the essential pieces of the puzzle you'll need to assemble to build a family through assisted reproduction. I'll discuss not only the people you will need by your side to help you create a baby but also the professionals who will help you navigate the process. We'll cover the basic science of sperm, eggs, embryos, conception, pregnancy, and birth. I'll discuss how donors and surrogates are screened, and how to choose one, and share stories of people I have helped through the process. I hope to show you that it is not only possible but also highly probable that you can become a parent through assisted reproduction if it's the path you choose.

Despite the growth of fertility resources, surrogacy and egg donor agencies, and a steadily increasing level of media attention on alternative families, assisted reproduction remains mysterious to most people. I travel the world talking about this issue and I'm asked the same basic questions over and over:

- Where do we start?
- How do we find reputable experts to help us?
- What are the legal issues we might be faced with?
- How do we put the biological pieces together?
- How do we tell our story to family, friends, and our child?

This book is designed to answer these and other commonly asked questions. However, my primary goal is not just to provide the nuts and bolts of assisted reproduction but also to share the human element of the process. Throughout the book I include real stories about people becoming parents, including those moments when things have gone well, times when they haven't, and some of the poignant moments that people have experienced during the process. I hope to bring the scientific, medical, and legal information to life, helping you to be educated and encouraged while keeping your expectations realistic.

This book will provide an introduction—a primer on assisted reproduction. It's a foundation on which you can build through additional books and resources that I've included at the end of the book. I'll cite some research where I think it can put your mind at ease and give you some ideas for further reading, but this book is by no means a comprehensive review. I leave that to my academic colleagues. Instead, I have drawn on my years of experience helping build families.

I have been helping people become parents my entire career as a psychologist. For over twenty years, I have specialized in the areas of parenting by choice and assisted reproduction at Growing Generations, an agency dedicated to making assisted reproduction easier, safer, and more gratifying for everyone involved. I have worked with all types of families: gay and lesbian couples, heterosexual couples dealing with medical conditions, infertility, and/or an inability to carry a child to term, single people who want to have a child, and even HIV-positive individuals.

I have written this book to help anyone who is contemplating having a baby with the help of others. It's also for family members, friends, employers, neighbors, and anyone else who knows someone who is either contemplating or building a family through third-party assisted reproduction. In particular, grandparents, aunts, and uncles will find this book useful as it both explains the basic process and helps one talk about it with other people.

Society has made great strides in overcoming bigotry, especially recently, but confusion and ignorance still breed hatred. The vast majority of the world's population is confused by or ignorant about alternative methods of procreation. This can lead to misunderstanding and judgment, which can affect how policies and legislation dealing with assisted reproduction are created. Creating families through ART is beautiful and healthy. It is about love, collaboration, and a desire to raise a child.

I love being a mom. It's the one thing that I always knew I wanted. I was one of those little girls who played with baby dolls, naming them and planning their futures, and even their children's futures. When I met and fell in love with my wife, Natalie, my wish to be a mother didn't go away, even though I knew there was never going to be a man in the picture. I always knew that I would be able to fulfill my dream of becoming a mommy. Thanks to a sperm donor, my wish came true.

When my daughters, Abby and Jenna, were born, it was rare for lesbians to have a baby. My kids are, essentially, the first generation of children born to LGBTQ parents. Natalie and I were in the vanguard. We learned a lot along the way. As a licensed psychologist, I realized what an advantage I had because I understood the importance of open, honest communication, support, trust, and flexibility, and it is this understanding that I bring to my work and that I offer to you in these pages.

Are You Ready?

If you've been thinking about becoming a parent, reading this book could flip a switch that pushes you forward toward your goal. I'll warn you now: once that switch is flipped, there's no going back. When Natalie and I had our first conversation about possibly starting the process of donor insemination and becoming parents, the switch flipped and we were in. Period. End of discussion. From that moment on, nothing was going to stop us.

When our first insemination attempt didn't take, we tried again. And when that didn't work, we tried again. And then we switched donors, thinking maybe different sperm would help. And when that didn't work, we tried again. And again. And then we switched donors again. We kept at it until finally, at last, I got pregnant with Abby. But never did we doubt that I would get pregnant and that we would be parents. We had decided that no matter what, we were going to be parents.

I see this same "flipping of the switch" all the time. A person or a couple will come to me for an initial consultation and say, "We're just looking into this, we're not ready right now, but maybe in a year or two we will be. At the moment, we're just gathering information." Then I'll get a call a week later because the switch flipped and all systems are go. The urgency kicks in full force, as something that previously felt unattainable now feels within reach. The possibility of parenthood becomes a reality.

You Can Build a Family, No Matter What

There is nothing more rewarding than building a family, and these days almost anyone can do so. The barriers that existed as few as ten or twenty years ago no longer stand in your way. If you are truly committed and you are willing to be patient, your wish can come true.

I must warn you, however, that having a baby through assisted reproduction is a marathon, not a sprint. You've got twenty-six miles to run, and no two miles are the same. And the marathon starts long before you start the race. You've got a whole lot of planning, training, and commitment ahead of time. You have to keep your eyes on the finish line even when things are really tough. Some miles are easy, others are excruciating, some are euphoric, and some are boring. That's exactly how having a baby through assisted reproduction feels. You plan, you put the pieces together, and you learn all you can about the process. There is a lot of waiting, anticipating, excitement, and sometimes disappointment. It proceeds in fits and starts, and sometimes you wonder if you'll ever see the finish line. But then, when you finally get there, it's the greatest thing ever. So, if you think you might be ready to take the first step, read on.

Chapter One

Getting Started

M ARCY AND ERIC had been trying to have a baby for several years with no luck. They'd been to many specialists and they'd tried everything their doctor suggested, without success. When their doctor finally suggested they explore surrogacy, rather than feeling excitement, they felt sad, ashamed, and hopeless. It was another six months before they called me and asked to talk about surrogacy. I met with them on and off for another six months while we explored their feelings of sadness and loss. Marcy especially needed to dig deep to uncover how she was feeling and to grapple with her excitement about being a mom in the context of what she would have to give up to get there. They eventually decided to proceed, and their surrogate, Annie, got pregnant on the first try. The pregnancy and delivery went smoothly, and Annie delivered a healthy baby girl. Still, every step of their process was fraught with sadness, loss, and regret. Until their baby was in their arms. From that moment on, they focused completely on the joy of raising their daughter. In an instant, the sorrow of their past was a distant memory.

Like Marcy and Eric, you may have some big emotional hurdles to overcome before you begin the process.[1] But with the support of professionals, family, and friends, and by staying focused on the outcome—your future family—you will get there.

Sometimes couples embrace the idea of getting help from the start, once they realize it is the only viable option, and even enjoy the process. For others, picking up this book is exciting and joyful, because you are setting a plan in motion to realize your dream of becoming a parent. Regardless of where you are emotionally, there is no shame about needing assistance, no sense of failing at something, but rather a sense of hope and possibility.

Note:

Assisted reproductive technology (ART) is by definition assisted. That means other people are involved in the process of conceiving a child. Before delving into the particulars of the medical options and procedures, and the various pieces you will need to put in place, it's important to determine if building a family this way is the right path for you.

Different readers of this book will be in very different places emotionally and psychologically. If you've tried to conceive a child naturally and haven't had success, it's likely you're feeling some grief about that fact. For you, exploring assisted reproduction may feel as if you've failed at something everyone else can do without much trouble. You may feel as if something is deeply and inherently wrong with you, and now you must take this unusual path to become a parent. When you understand that to realize your dream of parenthood you might have to give something up—one or even both of your genetic contributions, and/or the ability to carry and give birth to your baby—the emotional and psychological impact is undeniable. Why me? You might ask. While I can't answer that question, I can tell you that your feelings are totally valid. And after twenty years of experience helping prospective parents through third-party assisted reproduction, I know that if you truly want to become a parent and you choose assisted reproduction, you will eventually come to embrace it.

There are many, many people who have a child in a nontraditional way, but if you think there is something wrong with or shameful about having a child through assisted reproduction, then you shouldn't do it. A shred of doubt or uneasiness can grow. You are using exceptional means to bring a life into the world, and you need to be completely sure where you stand. Otherwise your choices can affect your ability to parent, your relationship with your child, and your relationship with your partner if you have one. If you feel embarrassed, or if you have moral or ethical concerns, then it is important to sort those out before you begin. Sometimes just a few conversations with a mental health professional can really help. Often, just talking through all of your feelings, understanding where they come from and having the opportunity to express and process your grief, can help you work through your feelings and then make a powerful choice. If after all of these conversations and research you are still uncomfortable with enlisting the help of others to have your family, you should choose a different option. There are many children in the world in need of loving parents, and fostering and adoption are wonderful ways to build a family. Being aware of where you're at emotionally, spiritually, and financially is an important first step in the process, and I encourage you to take a moment to check in with yourself and your partner if you have one. This is one of the most important decisions one can make, and the more facts you have about the process, and the more in tune you are with how you feel about your options, the easier it will be to make the decision that's right for you and your family.

The (Potential) Puzzle Pieces

There are four key players in your assisted reproduction journey:

- A medical specialist, your reproductive endocrinologist
- A reproductive attorney
- A mental health professional specializing in fertility and ART
- A fertility insurance expert

While some hopeful parents choose to go it alone, or go it partially alone (enlisting the help of a few but not all of these people), I would advise against that. For a life decision as major as this one, you'll want all the support you can get. And it's very likely that at some point you will need—yes, need—these experts to guide you through the legal, medical, and psychological aspects of third-party assisted reproduction. With that strongly worded advice out there, let's dive into how these four professionals can help you on your journey.

A Medical Specialist

Assisted reproduction can help you conceive a baby using your own sperm, eggs, and womb, with the fertilization process managed and guided by a reproductive endocrinologist, a highly specialized medical doctor. Reproductive endocrinologists are trained and certified as an obstetrician/gynecologist (OB/GYN) and then as a specialist in reproductive endocrinology, which is the science of reproduction. These are the doctors that help people get pregnant.

Fact: The American Society for Reproductive Medicine (ASRM) is a hub for reproductive endocrinologists and all other professionals in the field of ART and is a great resource for hopeful parents. An especially helpful tool is their collection of statistics online about how likely each reproductive endocrinologist is to help their patient get pregnant.

Reproductive endocrinologists are highly trained medical professionals. That said, just like any doctor, they have different personalities, different bedside manners, and different ways of working with patients. It's imperative that you find one you're comfortable with because this is a very intimate and emotional process. To this end, most are willing to have an initial consultation to go over their protocols, to talk about their statistics, and to discuss their overall approach. Before you commit to working with a specific doctor, it is wise to take advantage of this. If you can talk to a few former patients as well, even better.

When you visit a reproductive endocrinologist, you should expect a head-to-toe analysis of you and your partner. One important element of this will be blood work with the intended mother to look at hormone levels and similar issues that may be preventing pregnancy, and sperm analysis with the intended father to check for problems there. Often, after this assessment, the doctor will offer advice about timing sexual intercourse to maximize the potential for pregnancy and may suggest lifestyle changes to increase the odds of pregnancy, such as eating better, reducing stress, etc. If the intended mother's lab work indicates a need, she may be put on some type of fertility drug.

Often, this is enough to help a couple to get pregnant. When it's not, the likely next steps are insemination or IVF, or in vitro fertilization. With insemination, the doctor puts the intended father's sperm into the intended mother via catheter, in the ideal spot at the ideal time, to see if nature will take it from there. With IVF, eggs are removed from the intended mother, fertilized in a lab using the intended father's sperm, and nurtured to the embryo stage. Then the embryo is transferred back into the intended mother. I will discuss these processes in detail a bit later.

A reproductive endocrinologist can help you figure out why you can't get pregnant and what to do about it. Most of the time, some combination of timing, lifestyle, fertility drugs, insemination, and IVF results in pregnancy. If these options fail repeatedly, the doctor may suggest third-party assisted reproduction, which involves contributions from one or more third parties, like a sperm donor, an egg donor, or a gestational surrogate. The more people involved in your process of conceiving, carrying, and having your baby, the more complicated that process becomes. This is when other pieces—a lawyer, a mental health professional, insurance, financing, sperm donor, egg donor, and/or a surrogate—are essential to complete the puzzle. In these cases, you need to enlist the services of a lawyer and a psychologist, or an assisted reproduction agency, which will provide you with the legal, psychological, and medical expertise you need.

A Reproductive Attorney

If you need an egg donor or a surrogate, you need the services of a lawyer who specializes in reproductive law.

With egg donors and surrogates, there are specialized, incredibly detailed contracts. These contracts are designed to cover every aspect and potential aspect of the process, and to protect your rights as the intended parent. You need a good lawyer to make sure the contracts are meticulous and handled correctly. And that attorney needs to be a highly trained and experienced expert—so kindly decline your tax attorney uncle's offers to save you money and do the legal work for you for free.

If you're using a surrogate, your lawyer will help you make sure your surrogate lives in a surrogacy-friendly state—a state where surrogacy is legal and your rights as an intended parent are protected by statutes and case law. There are states where surrogacy is not legalized and your rights are not protected, and the consequences of attempting surrogacy in one of those states can be dire. This issue is discussed more fully later in the book, but it's worth mentioning here, too.

Your lawyer will also help you do whatever is necessary to establish your parental rights. If you're a same-sex couple, for instance, you may need to jump through a few extra hoops to make sure that both of you are the legal parents of your child. (This can be true even in some surrogacy-friendly states.) And, once again, different states have different laws and requirements, so you need a specialist lawyer to guide you and make sure that everything is planned ahead of time and done by the book.

Do not skimp on this part of the process. You will not be able to navigate this nuanced legal process on your own, and failing to get everything done correctly right from the start can be disastrous. I've listed useful information about lawyers who do this work in the Resources section.

A Mental Health Professional

Having the support of a mental health professional specializing in fertility and ART to help you through the process is not just a luxury; it is essential. As I mentioned earlier, you may be grieving the loss of the picture you had in your mind of how your family would come to be. A qualified mental health professional can help you work through your feelings and make the best choice for moving forward. He or she can help you navigate the unique relationship and feelings that may come up throughout the process of assisted reproduction, especially when third parties are involved.

Should you use a surrogate, your relationship with her will be unlike any you have ever had—it will involve a very strange intimacy with someone who may start out as a total stranger, or may be someone you already have a very different kind of relationship with. A psychologist will help you know what to anticipate as the relationship unfolds. A mental health professional will also screen all the parties involved to ensure transparency and lay the groundwork so that the process is set up for success. He or she will help educate all parties and set realistic expectations.

An agency that specializes in assisted reproduction will provide you with this service, but if you think you might go about it on your own, be sure to seek a qualified, experienced mental health provider. The ASRM can help you find an expert in this field.

A Fertility Insurance Expert

Assisted reproduction requires many types of insurance as you move through the process. If you're using your own sperm, eggs, and womb, your insurance may or may not help you get pregnant. If you're serious about beginning the process, one of the first phone calls you make should be to your insurance company to find out exactly what your coverage is. Some insurance companies will cover only part of your fertility treatments. Once you get pregnant, your insurance should cover you because it's your own pregnancy, but it's good to find out ahead of time just what your insurance covers.

If you need a third-party participant, especially if you need a surrogate, insurance gets considerably more complicated and expensive. First and foremost, you need specialized insurance that covers a surrogate pregnancy, or, at the very least, you need to make sure your surrogate has insurance that covers a surrogate pregnancy. Sometimes it will, but usually not. You also need special insurance that covers both the egg donor and the surrogate in the event of medical complications they might experience as they are going through the process. There are insurance agencies that specialize in this type of work, and I have listed them in the Resources section. Insurance costs can vary greatly. For example, cycle insurance, which covers egg donors and surrogates, is just a few hundred dollars, while pregnancy care insurance can range from $15,000 (if you are able to use the surrogate's own insurance, as you will pay her premium, deductible, and copays) to $30,000 if you need to buy the specialized surrogacy insurance.

Fact: Make sure your cycle and prenatal care insurance is in place *before* your surrogate becomes pregnant, as pregnancy is considered a preexisting condition, and the pregnancy and delivery can be very expensive without insurance.

Financing

Assisted reproduction, with or without third-party involvement, is very expensive. If you're working with a reproductive endocrinologist and attempting IVF, you can expect to spend upwards of $15,000 to $20,000 per cycle. If you need an egg donor as part of that process, the cost rises by around $50,000. If you need a surrogate, you're looking at another $120,000. Looking at the most expensive option—assisted reproduction with an egg donor and surrogate—it's likely that your total bill could be between $150,000 and $250,000 for one child. And most of that is out of pocket.

One of the variables that accounts for the range in cost is how many pregnancy attempts you need. Each additional embryo transfer costs around $20,000—for the medical bill, medication, and surrogate's travel to the clinic. When using an embryo created with an egg donor (so they have been tested and are healthy), surrogates are pregnant on the first try about 70 percent of the time, with the other 30 percent needing one or two more tries. Ninety-nine percent of surrogates will be pregnant within three tries. So most of the time intended parents will not have to pay for more than one embryo transfer. Still, the process is very expensive.

This should not be surprising when you think about everyone involved in the process. First, you've got a group of highly specialized professionals, and they get paid accordingly. Then you have people who contribute the biological requirements, and they too must be compensated. All the pieces of the puzzle come with a cost, and those costs are significant. It's also important to weigh the emotional cost of spending so much money on something that is not a sure thing. Is it worth going into debt to attempt to have a baby this way with no guarantee? Luckily, some surrogacy agencies are now offering guaranteed programs—there is no avoiding that you'll spend a lot of money, but they will stick with you until you have a baby. Still, the stress and pressure of the expense are worth exploring before you begin.

There are a few companies that will help you with the expenses by financing parts of the process, and there are also organizations that provide grants and scholarships. Lastly, almost every professional I know working in this field does at least a small amount of pro bono or sliding scale work, so you can always inquire about that. There are some options to help you manage the financial costs, but there is no denying that they are significant.

Assisted Reproduction Agencies

As you've no doubt come to realize, there are a lot of moving parts in building a family with assistance. At times, it can feel like you're herding kittens. It takes a lot of time and effort to line everything up properly and manage the process. If you enjoy herding kittens (and some people do), you can find the necessary professionals and manage the process yourself. Just make sure that you cover all the aspects I've discussed.

If the thought of herding kittens gives you hives, you can hire an agency to manage the process for you. Agency fees are typically between $20,000 and $40,000 (and they are included in the total cost that I mentioned above). That may seem expensive, but with an agency by your side, you have someone who's been through the process many times, who works with a knowledgeable and experienced group of professionals that provides thorough screenings for egg donors and surrogates before recommending them, and who knows how to handle whatever problems may arise. Wherever you are in your process, a good agency is always willing to have an initial conversation about what you need, what they provide, and what it will cost. And this initial conversation should be free. At the very least, this conversation can help educate you about the process.

Hiring an assisted reproduction agency is similar to hiring a contractor to build a house. When you decide to build a new home, you may want to work with an expert who can help you hire the best subcontractors and who knows the potential pitfalls you might face and how to best overcome them. Think about all the things involved: the architect, the cement company, the builder, the plumber, the electrician, the roofer, and the painter, plus all the permits and inspections required—not to mention all the snags you might encounter along the way. All of these things go into building a house. The only difference is who organizes and supervises the work. Just as you're not likely to know or understand all of the legal and logistical nuances in building a house, you are not likely, without assistance, to know or understand the legal and logistical nuances of third-party assisted reproduction. In addition, working with an agency will provide you with a type of advocate—someone you can turn to who will not only help you with the logistics and details that this process will entail but will also provide support, confidence, and a safety net as you go through the journey.

Now that we've laid the foundation, we can move on to the science of making a baby through assisted reproduction—the biological piece of the puzzle you need to create your future family. So here comes the good stuff.

CHAPTER TWO

Sperm

IN THE NEXT few chapters, I'll be doing a little refresher on your middle school sex education. (Who's in for a reprise of *The Miracle of Life*? Anyone?) We'll be going through the basics of male and female anatomy of the reproductive tracts, as well as introducing some of the key scientific terms used by assisted reproduction professionals. You may think you remember all this going in, but many (maybe even most) of my clients are missing some big facts in this area. Understanding what success looks like, and the myriad ways we can get there, is so important. So let's make sure we're all on the same page from the get-go.

The Basic Science of Sperm

Generally speaking, to make a baby we need three things—a male gamete (sperm), a female gamete (egg), and a uterus (womb) for the baby to grow in. In this chapter, I will primarily discuss the male gamete: sperm. I'll focus on eggs and the womb in chapters three and four.

First a bit of reproductive background: When a sperm and egg come together, the sperm penetrates the outer layer of the egg, fertilizing it. The fertilized egg is called a zygote until it begins to divide. After cell division begins, we call it an embryo. Within a few days of fertilization, the embryo implants in the womb, from which it draws nourishment. In the ninth week, give or take a few days, when the embryo has developed to a certain point, we refer to it as a fetus. As the fetus grows it looks more and more like a baby, both inside and out, until eventually, somewhere around the nine-month mark, a baby is born.

So sperm are important if you want to have a baby. Without sperm, an egg cannot be fertilized and a baby cannot be born.

Fact: Although women stop releasing eggs after menopause, men can produce and release sperm from puberty to death. This means that men have a much longer period of fertility than women do.

The process of generating and delivering sperm is relatively straightforward. Essentially, when puberty kicks in, a man's testicles (also known as testes) start producing sperm. At the same time, a pair of nearby glands—the seminal vesicle and the prostate—creates milky secretions that nurture and promote survival of the sperm. The combination of sperm and milky fluid that men ejaculate during orgasm (and slightly before and after orgasm) is known as semen. Typically, when men ejaculate, they release anywhere from 100 million to 200 million sperm.

Sperm are the smallest cells in the human body, approximately 1/100,000th of an inch in diameter. When viewed under a microscope, sperm look like tiny tadpoles, with a rounded head, a small midsection, and a long tail. The rounded head contains the man's genetic contribution to a future child (the man's chromosomes). The midsection holds fuel for the tail. The tail propels the cell through both the male and female reproductive tracts, helped along by muscle contractions within those regions. The head of the sperm is tipped by a thin layer of enzymes that break down the outer wall of a woman's egg, thereby allowing the sperm to penetrate and deliver its genetic payload. This layer of enzymes is called the acrosome.

When a baby is conceived through heterosexual intercourse, the man inserts his penis into a woman's vagina until he ejaculates. At that point, the man's sperm are still several inches away from the woman's egg. This is where the tail gets really busy, pushing the sperm upward in the woman from her cervix to her fallopian tubes. It's a long journey, and typically only a few hundred sperm ever get anywhere near the woman's egg.

If and when a sperm does reach the egg, the acrosome releases the enzymes that break the egg's shell, and the head of the sperm enters, leaving its midsection and tail behind. (The egg is only interested in the genetic portion of the sperm.) Once the sperm is in, the egg automatically creates an impermeable outer shield that repels all other sperm. And now we have a zygote—a fertilized egg that might, if we are lucky, grow into an embryo, and then a fetus, and then a baby.

Sperm and Potential Problems

There are all sorts of things that can go wrong with the spermatozoic portion of the baby-making process. First, there might be a problem with the sperm itself. Second, there might not be a man to provide the needed sperm. Third, once in a great while, often inexplicably, a man's perfectly healthy sperm and a woman's perfectly healthy egg just aren't compatible. So, no matter how hard they try, they just can't seem to make a baby.

The first of these issues, male infertility, arises for any number of reasons. Blockage of sperm ducts (usually the result of an STD or a vasectomy) is a relatively common cause. Another common cause is a varicocele, a collection of dilated veins near the testes that increases the region's temperature, thereby hindering the production of healthy sperm. (To produce healthy sperm, the temperature in the scrotum must be lower than the rest of the body.) Certain drugs and chemicals in the environment can also inhibit the production of healthy sperm, as can hormonal issues. And some men, for a variety of reasons, produce antibodies that destroy or incapacitate their sperm. There's a lot that can go wrong.

When couples are trying to conceive without success, the easiest variable to test is sperm. Standard sperm analyses, measuring sperm count, motility, and morphology (form and structure), have been around for many decades. Early on, sperm were analyzed under a microscope. Nowadays, the analysis is computer assisted and more accurate. Obvious problems like lack of sperm, poor swimmers, and deformed sperm are easily detected, but other issues are much harder to spot.

Some of these issues can be corrected via surgery or medications, while others cannot. But even the ones that can't be fixed with surgery or medication can usually be worked around. For instance, poor swimmers can be dealt with through in vitro fertilization (IVF), where an egg and a semen sample are placed in contact in a petri dish. So instead of the man's microscopically tiny and swim-challenged spermatozoa having to travel several inches inside a woman's reproductive tract to find the egg, they're placed at the vestibule, meaning all they must do is knock on the door and wriggle inside. And if that doesn't work, a single sperm can be captured and injected directly into an egg through a process known as intracytoplasmic sperm injection

(ICSI). IVF and ICSI also work well when low sperm count or sperm antibodies cause male infertility, as long as the morphology results are normal.

Even the blockage of sperm ducts can be overcome with testicular sperm extraction (TESE) or testicular sperm aspiration (TESA). Both processes are simple, safe, economical, and relatively painless. With TESE and TESA, sperm is pulled directly from the testes or a sperm duct using a very thin needle. Then, using the extracted sperm, an egg can be fertilized via IVF or ICSI.

Amazingly, even HIV-positive men can generate usable sperm, made safe through a "sperm washing" process. Since HIV pathogens live outside the sperm, not within it, a sperm sample can be chemically washed, removing the HIV pathogens. Once cleaned, the sperm can be used to fertilize an egg via IVF or ICSI, with virtually no risk of HIV to the woman who is going to carry the baby. Quite frankly, this process is amazing, and the pioneering work that I have had the honor to be a part of in this regard is, without doubt, one of the things I am most proud of.

One of my clients, Mark, created embryos with the help of an egg donor and was getting ready to transfer them into his surrogate. The week before the transfer, Mark tested HIV positive. He called me, devastated, thinking that he could never become a father. He didn't know that some forward-thinking doctors had developed a method that makes it safe for HIV-positive men to have their own genetic children. In fact, heterosexual couples had been safely using this procedure for a couple of years. It made total sense to use the sperm washing method with HIV-positive gay men, too. Mark couldn't use the embryos he'd created before his HIV-positive diagnosis, but with sperm washing he was able to create new embryos using his own sperm. Mark's baby girl was born two years after he found out he was HIV positive. His HIV status delayed the process, to ensure everything was completely safe for the surrogate and the baby, but he was still able to have his own genetic child.

Not all women are comfortable helping an HIV-positive man become a father, even when they understand and agree that the process is safe for them and the baby. And that's okay. There are plenty of women willing to do it. At Growing Generations, we've helped bring over one hundred babies into the world using sperm from dads who happen to be HIV positive.

Sperm Donation

Unfortunately, even though there are some amazing techniques available, sometimes a particular man's sperm just doesn't get the job done. Or, as mentioned above, there is not a man to provide the needed sperm. In these situations, sperm donation is a viable and available option.

Sperm can be donated directly—from a known donor to a known recipient—or through a sperm bank—where the donor is anonymous. Intended mothers are inseminated with donated sperm and fertilization can take place. The procedure usually happens in the doctor's office. Essentially, the reproductive endocrinologist injects the donated sperm into the woman's reproductive tract using a catheter, and then nature takes its course. In more complicated situations, eggs can be removed from the intended mother or an egg donor, fertilized via IVF or ICSI, and then transferred into the intended mother or a surrogate.

A Bit of History

The basic donor insemination process has been around for quite a while. In fact, the first reported instance of sperm donation and assisted insemination occurred in 1884 when Professor William Pancoast of Philadelphia's Jefferson Medical College inseminated the wife of a sterile merchant using sperm from one of his students. Unfortunately, this procedure was done in front of Dr. Pancoast's class without the woman's or even her husband's knowledge and consent.

It seems that Dr. Pancoast had been treating the couple for infertility for several months, eventually concluding that the issue was low sperm count in the husband. So he invited the wife in for yet another examination, chloroformed her, and had his class vote on which student was best-looking. That student then provided Dr. Pancoast a sperm sample, and nine months later the woman gave birth to a healthy baby boy. The incident was not reported publicly until 1909, twenty-five years after the fact, when the handsome student, now a doctor in his own right, published a confessional letter in a well-known medical journal.[1]

Super creepy, right? And not how we do things today.

As the 1900s progressed, doctors began to perform private donor inseminations relatively regularly. But they kept the practice quiet. Typically, they kept no records of these procedures so that donors (usually the doctors themselves, or members of their staff) could not be sued for child support. By the 1950s the situation had changed significantly. Doctors were performing the procedure openly, typically using frozen sperm samples, and the process was written about in numerous medical journals. Today, sperm donation is common.

Most sperm donors are college students. In fact, sperm banks are often located on or very near college campuses. For instance, there are sperm banks in Westwood (UCLA), Berkeley (UC Berkeley), Palo Alto (Stanford), and Cambridge (Harvard and MIT). Sometimes a sperm bank will have collection facilities at multiple universities. Usually they recruit with advertisements in campus publications such as, "Sperm donors needed to help infertile couples have babies. Compensated for your time."

Typically, sperm donors are not thinking at all about being parents. They just want to make a few quick bucks (anywhere from a few hundred to a few thousand dollars for a series of donations, depending on how many donations are made). Sure, there might be a little bit of altruism in some cases, but usually a sperm donor is just a young man looking for a bit of easy money, no strings attached. By donating to a sperm bank or doctor's office, the donor legally gives up any rights or responsibilities to any future offspring conceived using his sperm. If a donor makes a direct deposit (not through a bank or doctor's office) such as with a known donor, no such legal protections exist and the parents need to consult a reproductive attorney to have a contract with the donor stipulating his rights, responsibilities, and roles—or lack thereof.

The process of donating sperm is straightforward. The donor goes into a room with a sterile collection cup. Usually the sperm bank has placed porn in the room, either magazines or a laptop with videos. Then the donor does his thing, seals the collection cup, and turns it over to a staff member. It's all very sexy and glamorous.

If a donor doesn't want to handle things manually, some facilities have a machine called a sperm extractor. Sperm extractors are, well, hilarious. Basically, they're machines that give sperm donors (or whoever else is interested) an electronic hand job—with adjustable height, temperature, and pull frequency to make the experience more enjoyable. There is even a small video screen to help users get in the mood.

The Screening Process

Initial screening for sperm donors is pretty straightforward. The sperm bank first collects basic information about the man, like his height, weight, and level of education. Then the donor fills out a brief questionnaire asking about his personal and family history, including whether there is a history of cancer, depression, bipolar disorder, or other conditions among family members. Then there is a blood test to check for HIV, STDs, and other obvious medical issues. The sperm is also analyzed for sperm count, motility, and morphology.

In addition to sperm and blood testing, some sperm banks do psychological testing, such as a basic personality test. Sometimes they even obtain verified SAT scores, as intelligence is important to many people in the market for sperm. A reputable and well-established sperm bank will go beyond the basic screening and carry out these additional tests. The purpose of all this testing is twofold: to ensure the sperm is as healthy as possible from a medical standpoint so it is most likely to lead to a healthy baby, and to provide as much information about the donor to the intended parents as possible so they can make an informed choice.

Choosing a sperm donor is a very personal process. For some couples, matching the characteristics of the parent whose genetics are not in the mix is the most important thing. For others, avoiding certain characteristics takes precedence. Hair and eye color, height, ethnicity, education, hobbies, interests, and character traits are all factors to be considered.

Parents can pick up the sperm from the bank and literally drive it over to the fertility doctor (it comes frozen in a tiny vial in a large nitrogen tank that keeps it cold), or it can be shipped directly to the doctor's office. Some daring parents have done home inseminations, but this is definitely not something you should do if you don't have the medical expertise. Once the sperm is at the doctor's office, the doctor will thaw it out and inject the sperm via catheter into the mom's reproductive tract around the time that she is ovulating. With unprotected intercourse each cycle has a 25 percent chance of resulting in pregnancy when everything is working perfectly, so it's normal for insemination to take a few months to be successful. If it doesn't work the first time, you can try again the next month. There are pretty sophisticated ovulation tests, and many doctors will also use an ultrasound to check the timing. If you've tried insemination for months and it hasn't resulted in a pregnancy, your doctor might recommend adding fertility drugs to increase egg development and release. If that doesn't work, the doctor will likely recommend IVF or ICSI, which are discussed in detail in the next chapters. Sperm is prepared differently before it is frozen for insemination versus IVF, so you'll want to make sure you purchase the right formula. Your doctor and sperm bank will help with this.

Fact: Urban legend has it that male sperm swim faster, but female sperm are sturdier. So the timing of insemination can impact the sex of the baby. Inseminating right before ovulation is rumored to be more likely to result in a male baby, as the fastest swimmers will arrive first and fertilize the egg. For a girl, inseminating two or three days before ovulation may mean the sturdier female swimmers are still around when the egg is finally released. That said, nature often has other plans. And this is just legend, after all.

If you're using donated sperm, one important choice you must make is whether to use a known sperm donor (usually a friend or relative of the nonbiological parent) or an anonymous donor (usually found through a sperm bank). Both options have pros and cons.

One clear advantage with a known sperm donor is that you and your child will never have to wonder about their genetics. When your child asks, "Why do I have red hair?" you can point to your redheaded sperm donor friend and say, "You got that from him." Conversely, if you use an anonymous donor, and your child asks what their sperm donor was like and if they look like him, or if they have similar interests and personalities, you won't be able to answer in much detail.

A clear advantage of using an anonymous donor through a sperm bank is that you will not have the complication of someone you know wanting a role in your child's life that wasn't what you intended.

However, it's also important that you consider how your future child will feel about having access or not having access to their genetic contributors. While love makes a family, genetic links cannot be ignored. Some people now feel that using anonymous donors is unfair to the child, as they will not know half of their genetic makeup. Because of this, some professionals and agencies are moving more and more toward recommending open identity donors.

Whatever you decide, you need to thoroughly consider both options because you're going to have to explain the whole process to your child and possibly to a lot of other people— family members, friends, and even nosy neighbors who can't seem to stop themselves from asking well-intentioned but intrusive questions. So, when deciding between a known versus anonymous donor, consider the following:

- How am I going to manage other people's curiosity?

- What answers would I prefer to give?

- How do I want my child to see things as he or she grows up?

- Is it important to me that my child knows their donor?

- Will it be important to my child to know their donor? And is it fair for me to make that decision on their behalf?

- How will I feel if I can't provide my child with information about their donor?

- What will I do if my child wants to meet their donor?

- Do I have a man in my life who would be a good donor and who has the same expectations about the process as I do?

- What if my known donor wants more involvement than I want him to have? How will I navigate that?

If you use a known donor, such as a friend, sibling, or cousin, and he stays in your life, he may struggle with the idea that he is only a biological contributor and not the father. In fact, it's a rare individual who can be a known donor and not feel, at least a little bit, like a parent. And if the donor occasionally oversteps your healthy boundaries by inserting himself as a parent, it can be confusing to your child.

Regardless of whether your donor is known or anonymous, rest assured that you and your partner are the parents. Even if your sperm donor is a friend who remains in your child's life, you can reinforce that you are the parents. When explaining this to your child, you can say something like, "We wanted you very much, but we needed a part from a man that we didn't have to make that happen. Joe, who is a very good friend of ours and wanted to help us, gave us some of his sperm. And now we have you." You just need to make it crystal clear to your child, right from the start, that your donor is a donor and not a parent. He didn't give you his sperm because he wanted to become a parent; he did it so you could have a baby that you really, really wanted. Of course, if you did decide at the beginning that Joe will be a co-parent, then that's the truth that you relay to your child.

If you're truthful and clear from the start, your child will not be confused. And you will instill a sense of confidence and security in your child as you affirm your family. It is imperative to have clear conversations with all parties to set up expectations in advance. To this end, a mental health professional can be very helpful. If you are using a known donor, you will also need the help of a reproductive attorney, as you'll need a contract that will spell out everyone's expectations very clearly.

Sometimes people don't want to share the fact that they've used a donor. If you simply keep quiet, your family, friends, and pesky neighbors may assume you got pregnant the old-fashioned way. And your child will assume that too unless he or she is told the truth. However, I always vote for telling the truth, at least with your child. Research regarding sperm donation and disclosure to your child informs us that openness and honesty result in the best outcomes for kids. Uniformly telling the truth produces the healthiest kids. Even in situations where you can pass, it is my strong professional belief that it's better to go with the truth. And the sooner you start telling the truth, the better off you and your child will be.[2]

If you're a male couple, your sperm-related issues are primarily focused on which partner should provide the sperm. After all, only one man can be the biological contributor to one egg. Similarly, if you are a female couple, you'll be deciding which of you will be inseminated. Admittedly, technology is changing rapidly, and at some point gene splicing may progress to the point where DNA from two men could be combined and used to fertilize one egg, or DNA from two women could be spliced and then fertilized by one sperm. But for now this is not an option.

Sometimes the choice of whose sperm to use is an easy one—one of you may really want to use yours and the other doesn't care. Or maybe there is a family history of health issues, addiction, or mental illness on one side so you use the other. It is also possible to take sperm samples from both partners, mixing the semen together so you and your partner each have an equal chance of being the biological father. However, doctors typically don't like this approach and I don't recommend it either, as it's a bit more complicated medically, ethically, and legally.

In cases where both of you want to be a biological father, you can "take turns." Essentially, when you get a batch of eggs from your donor (usually around ten or twenty are harvested), you can fertilize half of the eggs with one partner's sperm and half of the eggs with the other partner's. Then you take a fertilized egg from one of you and put it in the surrogate, freezing the rest of the embryos for later use. After you have your first child, you can have another, this time using an embryo from the other father. Or, if you want twins (much more on twins later), you can use one embryo from each of you, transferring them at the same time. If one takes but the other doesn't, you can go back when you are ready and use an embryo from the other dad.

In cases where there will be two moms who both want to be genetic parents the idea is the same, although the logistics are different. You can use the donated sperm to inseminate one of you first, and then for a second child you can inseminate the other.

Whether you are a two-dad family using only one of your sperm, a two-mom family taking turns, or a family using a sperm donor, only one parent will be genetically linked to the child. It is really important that you sort through any feelings you may have about being a nonbiologically related parent before your baby is born. A mental health professional can be very helpful here, but the most important thing is that both parents are on the same page and acknowledge that they will both be full and equal parents regardless of biology.

Allen and Isaac, a legally married gay couple who'd been together for about ten years, both wanted to have a biological connection to their kids. When I explained that they could each fertilize half the eggs, and they could have a baby with their own genetics, they were thrilled. But they kept referring to the babies they were planning as "his baby" and "my baby." It was obvious they were struggling to believe that with any children they had they would be equal parents, regardless of genetics.

Eventually, Allen and Isaac decided to try for twins using one embryo fertilized by each father. However, one of the embryos didn't implant, so they only had one baby—from an egg fertilized by Allen. As soon as that beautiful baby girl was born, they started talking about having "Isaac's baby" next. They continued to struggle to believe that they were equal parents—not just to the baby they had, but to any they had in the future. They went on to have a son, and after he was born we had many conversations about their family of four and how much they both loved and felt connected to both children. Allen and Isaac eventually came to realize that their connection to their children went beyond biology.

No matter your situation, it's important that you understand and truly believe that you are both 100 percent the parent. When you are unified in this way, you send a message to the universe and the universe responds in kind. When people have questions, you can make it clear that you are both the parent, and that's how people will see it. If you want to then answer the question about who the biological contributor is, you can do so—but you don't have to. That is a very personal choice. Biology is not the determining factor in parenthood. It's love that makes a family, not genetics. So no matter where the sperm comes from—the dad, an anonymous sperm donor, or a friend—the parents are the parents.

CHAPTER THREE

Eggs

W E'VE DISCUSSED the male's genetic contribution, the sperm. Now let's take a look at the female's genetic contribution, the egg. I think a basic primer about the female reproductive system is important.

The female reproductive tract consists of, from the outside working in, the vulva, the vagina, the cervix, the uterus, the fallopian tubes, and the ovaries. The fallopian tubes are narrow cylinders about four inches in length, leading from the uterus to the ovaries. At the end nearest the ovaries are tiny fingerlike protrusions known as fimbriae, which find mature eggs, pulling them from the ovary walls and sending them down the tube for potential fertilization. The ovaries are walnut-size globular structures, one on each side, adjacent to the fimbriae. The ovaries have two important functions. First, they discharge certain hormones into the bloodstream. Second, and more important for our purposes here, they release eggs for procreation, a process referred to as ovulation.

Eggs, also known as ova or oocytes, are the largest cells in the human body, about the size of a powdery grain of sand. They are actually visible to the human eye without the aid of a microscope. On a monthly cycle (approximately), the ovaries select a few eggs for development and maturation. This occurs in tiny blister-like structures, known as follicles, which project from the surface of the ovaries. When an egg is ready, the fimbriae, or tiny "fingers" at the ovary end of the fallopian tubes, retrieve the egg with a vacuum-like process and direct it into and through the fallopian tubes for possible fertilization.

Fact: A woman develops all the eggs she will ever have by the fetal age of 12 weeks. At that time, she has approximately 7 million eggs and at birth she will have about 1 million eggs. By the time she hits puberty, she's down to about 300,000. She uses about 300 to 400 of those eggs during the approximately 400 ovulations that occur during her reproductive life span.

Human eggs are similar in structure to chicken eggs, though obviously on a much smaller scale. In the center of the egg (analogous to the yolk) is the nucleus, which carries the female's genetic material (her chromosomes). The surrounding ooplasm (the egg white), also known as cytoplasm, contains microorganelles, which supply energy for the egg and the embryo for a short while after fertilization, helping it grow before becoming attached to an external source of nourishment (the endometrium).

A Bit of History

Since before modern times scientists have tried to understand how human beings reproduce. Early on it was thought that a man's semen and woman's blood were involved. Based on studies of chickens, Aristotle posited that the mixture produced an egg in the uterus from which a baby developed. This idea lasted for nearly two thousand years until William Harvey disproved that idea when he looked at a number of animals right after mating and found that the female's uterus was empty—no egg to be found. He did, however, rightly propose that all creatures arise from eggs; they just had yet to be found in mammals. This led to an intensive search for the eggs in mammals and resulted in the discovery of the existence and role of the ovaries and fallopian tubes. The seventeenth century brought the microscope, and with it the ability to look more closely at semen and the sperm within. The mammalian egg remained undiscovered for another two hundred years, until 1826, when Karl Ernst von Baer discovered the ovum when looking at a dog ovarian follicle under a microscope. With the advent of cell theory in 1938 by Theodor Schwann and Matthias Jakob Schleiden it was recognized that the ovum was a cell, its nucleus was discovered, meiosis was described, and the role of the chromosomes in heredity was revealed.[1]

Eggs are very delicate compared to sperm, which are almost shockingly hardy. Sperm will stay alive in the cervix, womb, and/or fallopian tube for an amazingly long time—from two to seven days. Sperm will even stay alive outside the body for several hours before they're frozen. Moreover, they can be frozen and thawed without any problems. Eggs, however, have a very definite shelf life, and they can only be fertilized twelve to twenty-four hours after ovulation. This means there is only a small window every month when a woman can get pregnant.

Eggs and Potential Problems

As with sperm, there are all sorts of potential complications with eggs. First, there might be a problem with the production of eggs or the eggs that are produced. Or, as stated before, once in a great while a man's perfectly healthy sperm and a woman's perfectly healthy egg just aren't compatible.

The first of these issues, female infertility, arises for a number of reasons, the most common of which is damaged or blocked fallopian tubes that prevent the egg from uniting with sperm. Sexually transmitted diseases are a common cause of tubal scarring and blockage, as are various forms of pelvic surgery.

Damaged or nonfunctioning ovaries might also contribute to infertility. Sometimes an ovary cannot properly mature an egg due to hormonal issues. Sometimes an ovary cannot release an egg, even though hormonal levels are optimal and the egg is adequately developed. Other times eggs are trapped within the ovary due to scarring or a thickening of the ovary's surface. Women may also develop antibodies to their partner's sperm, preventing fertilization.

Abnormal ovulation is another cause for female infertility. Some women do not ovulate at all, while others ovulate too early or too late in their cycle for a pregnancy to occur. Age can play a role in this. As women age, ovulation is more likely to become abnormal. It is also believed that the quality of eggs diminishes as women get older. As such, female fertility typically wanes after the age of thirty-five.

Many of these issues can be overcome medically, often via surgical egg retrieval from the intended mother followed by fertilization via IVF or ICSI. If, however, an intended mother simply does not produce healthy and fully developed eggs, or if there is not a woman to provide the necessary egg, egg donation offers a viable solution.

Egg Donation

Today, egg donation is a common and medically safe practice available to anyone who needs help. Infertile heterosexual cou ples, fertile heterosexual couples who are worried about pass- ing on a genetically borne disease or some other genetic defect, single men, and gay men have all benefitted from this medical advancement.

In the United States, egg donation is governed by the Food and Drug Administration (FDA) and overseen by the American Society for Reproductive Medicine (ASRM). If you are inter- ested in reading these guidelines for yourself, you can find the link in the Resources section at the end of this book. What's more important than you knowing the specific guidelines is that you make sure your doctor, lawyer, mental health pro- vider, and/or agency are knowledgeable and choose to follow the guidelines.

Fact: The first reported case of a child being born from a donated egg was in Australia in 1983. The following year, the first US egg donation baby was born at UCLA Medical Center. Prior to this breakthrough, adoption was the only viable route to parenthood for single men, gay men, and many infertile couples.

Who Are Egg Donors, and Why Do They Do It?

Like sperm donors, egg donors tend to be college and/or graduate students, usually between twenty-one and twenty-nine years old. Much of the time they know someone who needs an egg donor, perhaps a relative or a neighbor, or they have a friend who donated and felt really gratified. So, unlike sperm donors, they're not answering ads tacked to the coffee shop bulletin board. It's much more personal than that. Egg donors say things like, "My uncle is gay and I know that he would be a great dad," "I read a story about egg donation, and it sounded really cool," or "my roommate donated her eggs and felt really good about herself afterward."

In general, egg donors are motivated by a mix of healthy ego and altruism. An egg donor might think, "My genes are great. I'm attractive. I'm smart. I'm an athlete. I'm musically gifted. I'm also young and don't want to have kids of my own for another decade or so. Meanwhile, every month I'm shedding these cells that are meaningless to me that other people really want. So maybe I can do some good by helping someone else become a parent."

Egg donors are paid a lot more than sperm donors, generally between $5,000 and $15,000 per donation. And egg donors absolutely should be paid more than sperm donors because egg donation involves a series of injections followed by a medical procedure with some risk, whereas sperm donation involves masturbation.

Egg donors are compensated for their effort, risk, time, and the overall inconvenience of donating, not for their gametes. The vast majority of egg donors, when they are properly screened, are interested in becoming donors because they are young, vibrant, intelligent, attractive women who feel good about their genes and want to help someone else. The financial reward is really just to compensate for the effort and inconvenience.[2]

The Screening Process

Potential egg donors should be screened very thoroughly. In a reputable clinic or agency only about 2 percent of egg donor applicants make it all the way through the screening and approval process.

Fact: The extensive egg donor screening is the opposite of what happens at most sperm banks, where almost any reasonably healthy male is accepted. Sperm donors show up, do their business, and are out. Meanwhile, egg donors go through a lengthy screening process before they can be approved. Science or sexism? You decide.

The screening process includes medical testing, genetic testing, psychological testing, sometimes intelligence testing, a criminal background check, and educational counseling. Intelligence testing is done because the intended parents are nearly always interested in that. The rest is medically and psychologically necessary to ensure that the donor is fully informed and consenting and that she is healthy enough for the process. Our screening process at Growing Generations is intensive, but we feel it's better to be safe than sorry, so we err on the side of caution.

For egg donors, there is no such thing as being a truly anonymous donor. Intended parents aren't given the egg donor's name, but they usually get pictures—baby pictures, pictures growing up, current pictures, and sometimes even video. And with constantly evolving facial recognition software, it is very easy to identify a person from a picture. So even though egg donors are technically anonymous, it's not total anonymity. One of the standard questions we ask donor applicants is, "How would you feel if twenty years from now someone knocked on your door and said, 'Hi, I think you were my egg donor?'" Because, in truth, there is a reasonable chance that will happen.

I get a range of responses to this question. Some women say, "That would be weird, but okay." Others say, "I think that would be kind of interesting and cool." Answers like that are fine, coming from an egg donor. But if a woman says, "That would be devastating, and I wouldn't like it at all," then she shouldn't be an egg donor. And she wouldn't pass our screening because we don't want her to do something she might later regret.

Egg donors often say they're perfectly willing to meet the intended parents, and to meet the offspring later if that is desired. Again, this is pretty much the opposite of sperm donation, where a man who donated three years ago has no idea if/when/how his sperm is being used. Egg donors absolutely know that they've been chosen and their eggs are being used, mostly because we don't harvest their eggs until we know for sure that somebody wants them.

Fact: More and more egg donor agencies differentiate between donors who are willing to meet the intended parents and the offspring and those who are not. Donors willing to meet intended parents and offspring are known as "open identity," "yes," "ID option," or "open release" donors. If this is important to you, make sure you choose one of these donors.

As egg freezing becomes more viable, egg banks, similar to sperm banks, where egg donors undergo the procedure and then their eggs are frozen and utilized at a later date, will be an option.

Again, most egg donors are not in it for the money. Most reputable agencies screen to assure this, because we don't want anyone to feel manipulated or exploited. So we make sure a potential donor understands the risks involved, that she will need to take fertility drugs via injections, and that harvesting the eggs is a medical procedure and has some risk, inconvenience, and discomfort. If she's willing to go through all of that *because she wants to do it*, and if she passes all the other screenings, then she is a good candidate.

Donor Caitlin says, "I have a friend who donated and I asked her about the process. Although it sounded physically challenging, I could tell that she found it to be a very rewarding experience. I liked the idea of getting to contribute to someone out there who will truly appreciate being able to start a family. For me, this just felt like living life to the fullest, and helping someone else do the same."

Another thing we talk about during the screening process is the need for each donor to have a support network. Donors need to communicate with their loved ones that they are donating eggs. Keeping it a secret is not recommended. Imagine on the morning of the egg retrieval the donor tells her mom she needs a ride to the doctor's office. Her mom asks why, and when her daughter tells her she is planning to donate eggs, the mother responds, "Over my dead body!" And suddenly the donor is backing out. To prevent last-minute changes of heart, we require that egg donors tell the important people in their life what they're planning to do. They need to have people supporting them emotionally and at times even physically. So if someone important in a donor's life is going to have a very negative reaction, we want to know that early on. At the very least, the donor needs someone to drive her home after the retrieval takes place. And of course we want this to be an experience that the donor is proud of and feels good about.

Egg Retrieval

Egg retrieval is a lengthy process. It begins with six to twelve weeks of hormonal regulation and stimulation, with a round of birth control to regulate the donor's cycle. First, the donor is put on birth control, which helps to control the timing of her reproductive cycle by controlling when menstruation will begin and, therefore, when controlled ovarian stimulation should begin. This can be important because some doctors like to implant "fresh" embryos (as opposed to frozen embryos), and for this the reproductive cycles of the egg donor and the person who is going to carry the embryo must be in sync. However, more and more doctors are doing frozen embryo transfers, so syncing the cycles is becoming less important.

Once the ovarian cycle is regulated to the fertility doctor's satisfaction, the egg donor is taken off birth control and placed on fertility drugs. There are two reasons for this. First, these drugs enhance the growth and development of the woman's ovarian follicles, increasing the number of mature (ready to harvest) eggs. A woman not on fertility medications usually produces either one or two mature eggs per cycle. With fertility medications, women typically produce ten to twenty mature eggs per cycle. Second, doctors can control the timing of ovulation in ways that allow them to surgically retrieve the eggs at full maturity, just a few hours before they would be discharged through ovulation.

Today, doctors typically rely on gonadotropins—hormones produced in the pituitary glands—to stimulate egg production. Gonadotropins lead to the secretion of estradiol—an estrogen steroid—and testosterone, which leads to secondary sex characteristics in both men and women, such as hair growth, muscle development, breast development, and voice change.

There are two commonly utilized gonadotropins: follicle stimulating hormone (FSH) and luteinizing hormone (LH). Because these drugs cannot be absorbed through digestion, they must be administered via injection. Typically, this process begins on day two or three of the ovarian cycle and ends between days eight and twelve of the cycle.

Doctors monitor egg development in donors via blood estradiol levels and ultrasound assessment, and when they feel the time is right, they will inject HCG (human chorionic gonadotropin), which finishes the egg maturation process and leads to ovulation and menstruation within thirty-eight to forty-two hours. At around the thirty-six-hour mark, shortly before the anticipated time of ovulation, the eggs are surgically retrieved.

Typically, egg retrieval is performed in the fertility doctor's office or in an outpatient surgery center. Usually, the procedure is performed under "conscious sedation," where the donor has an altered level of consciousness and doesn't remember the procedure but isn't totally "knocked out." As with any form of anesthesia, there are risks. But conscious sedation is significantly less dangerous than general anesthesia, where the patient is completely and totally unconscious.

The process of egg retrieval is straightforward yet delicate. The reproductive endocrinologist inserts a long ultrasound probe into the vagina. The probe sends images to a screen visible to the doctor, clearly showing the ovarian follicles. Guided by the ultrasound image, the doctor inserts a sterile needle through the vagina and into the ovarian follicles, gently sucking the eggs from the follicles and into the needle. Eggs can also be retrieved via laparoscopic surgery, going through a tiny incision in the naval or the pelvic cavity, but most doctors prefer ultrasound-guided needle retrieval.

Successful donor egg retrieval cycles typically yield ten to twenty eggs. Out of that group about 70 percent will fertilize, with about 50 percent of those yielding a chromosomally healthy embryo. So if you harvest ten mature eggs, you will likely end up with three or four healthy embryos, which is an excellent result.

The Waiting Game

The process of egg retrieval takes anywhere from six weeks to three months, and this can be one of the boring miles in the marathon. As mentioned above, there are a few weeks on birth control, and then one to two weeks of fertility drugs before retrieval. And before any of that occurs there are legal contracts to deal with. The donor has contracts, the intended parents have contracts, the insurance company has contracts, and the agency has contracts. None of these agreements are in any way contentious, but they still take time, and the medical process can't start until the paperwork is completely in order.

Unfortunately, after all this effort there are still occasions when you arrive at the retrieval and there are no eggs, or the donor ovulated sooner than expected, or the eggs that are harvested just don't look right. The doctors do a lot to mitigate this because they monitor the donor very closely, but retrievals can still be a bust.

Because eggs are delicate, they are typically fertilized immediately after being harvested. However, technology is changing rapidly, and harvested eggs can now be frozen for later use with a modicum of success. As of this writing, the success rate with frozen eggs is not as high as sperm, but technologies are being developed to remedy this.

Egg banking, or freezing eggs for later use, is enticing because it cuts out a lot of the waiting involved with egg retrieval as well as the risk that you won't get much for your efforts. Intended parents can purchase frozen eggs much the way sperm is purchased. As the efficacy of freezing and thawing eggs improves, egg banks will be more common.

In all likelihood, egg donors would also prefer egg banking. With the current system, after egg donors pass through our screening we create a profile for them and that profile goes on a website available to intended parents. Then, when an egg donor is chosen, the process begins. But until then, they're in limbo. With egg banking, a donor could start the retrieval process as soon as she passes the screening. Her eggs would be harvested and frozen within a few weeks—instead of a few months (or maybe even years)—and she'd get paid. It's likely the egg bank would pay a lower fee because there is no guarantee that the donor's eggs will be chosen and she wouldn't have to wait for payment;

but that payment would be a sure thing. It's a surer thing for parents too, because the eggs have already been retrieved.

Choosing Your Egg Donor

Like sperm donation, choosing your egg donor is something you should consider carefully. There are two basic types of egg donors: known donors (usually a family friend or an intended parent's sibling or family member) and anonymous donors (who, as discussed above, aren't nearly as anonymous as sperm donors can be).

Some people really want to use a known donor—especially if it's a family member, because they want to be closer genetically to their kids. This is perfectly fine, as long as the chosen donor actually wants to do it. But what I find is a lot of the time they don't. If you show up with your sister or a cousin or your best gal pal, I will talk to all of you together and everything might be fabulous. Then, a little bit later, I will get your potential donor alone in a room and the first thing she says is, "Please get me out of this. I don't want to do this, but I don't know how to say no without upsetting everyone." Then I facilitate a discussion where the person asked to donate can express how she truly feels.

If you are considering asking a family member or a friend to donate her eggs, it's important that you realize she may say yes under duress. Although she would like to help you, deep down she might have serious reservations about it but be afraid to tell you. A psychologist will work with you to ensure that all parties are on the same page. I can't express the importance of this enough. Complete honesty is key, because you do not want to force someone into doing something this important and have her resent it or regret it for the rest of her life.

If you do decide to use a known donor, she goes through all of the same screening as any other donor, plus an extra layer of screening where we talk about what it's like to have a biological connection to a child in her family or friendship group that's not her child. Your donor needs to think carefully about this, and about how she will feel watching this child grow up without having the say of a parent.

A known egg donor is likely to be a significant part of your life and your child's life. You need to be aware that this presents an extra layer of connection and potential complication, and fully consider how you will view and treat your donor moving forward.

With anonymous egg donors you don't have this extra layer of connection and potential complication. That does not, however, mean that one way is better than the other. Each intended parent is unique, with different values and goals, so each intended parent needs to decide what's best for his or her family. The important thing here, as with every aspect of ethical third-party assisted reproduction, is that everything is out in the open, fully explored, discussed, and consented to. As in the case when choosing a sperm donor, those same questions exist when choosing an egg donor. When deciding between a known versus anonymous donor, consider the following:

- How am I going to manage other people's curiosity?

- What answers would I prefer to give?

- How do I want my child to see things as they grow up?

- Is it important to me that my child knows their donor?

- Will it be important to my child to know their donor? And is it fair for me to make that decision on their behalf?

- How will I feel if I can't provide my child with information about their donor?

- What will I do if my child wants to meet their donor?

- Do I have a woman in my life who would be a good donor and who has the same expectations about the process as I do?

- What if my known donor wants more involvement than I want her to have? How will I navigate that?

Laura and Sam had been going through IVF treatment for over two years, after three years of trying on their own. They'd done six unsuccessful rounds of IVF, attempting to create their own genetic embryos to no avail. Their doctor advised them to turn to egg donation, but they felt strongly that they couldn't turn to an anonymous egg donor. It just didn't feel right to them. At the same time, Laura's older sister, Sarah, offered to be their donor. Sarah already had two children and felt very comfortable donating for her sister. Sam, Laura, Sarah, and Sarah's husband were counseled together and separately, and it was clear that their expectations aligned and that Sarah fully understood what she was getting into. The donation was successful, and Laura and Sam were able to create embryos using Sarah's eggs and Sam's sperm. An embryo was transferred into Laura and she got pregnant on the first try. Sarah and Laura's kids know about their special connection but see themselves as the cousins that they are.

If you opt for an anonymous egg donor, you will have your own unique factors and criteria that influence who you choose. You might want certain physical traits, or a certain level of intelligence. You may want the donor to be an athlete, or a musician, or good at math and science. You may want a certain ethnicity, usually to match your own, but not always. Or maybe that's not important at all.

Chris and Mike were searching for a donor. Chris is African American, and Mike is a redheaded Caucasian. They kept sending me, separately, pictures of donors who looked like their partner. They were planning for twins, with one embryo fertilized by each man, but each wanted the egg donor to look like his partner. It was adorable. I told them they were obviously a match made in heaven, because what they were attracted to, even in an egg donor, was the same as what they were attracted to in a partner. They ended up finding the perfect donor, a mixed-race woman who looked a little like both of them, and had twins—a boy and a girl—that resembled their parents.

Sometimes the information that you base your decision on turns out to be not that important in the long run. For instance, when Natalie and I first started looking for a sperm donor, we opted for a Jewish donor because we're both Jewish. We thought that's what we wanted. We tried with his sperm three times and didn't get pregnant. So we obtained another donor's sperm. This man was less like us in some ways, and more like us in others. But we couldn't get pregnant with his sperm, either. Finally, we told the sperm bank that we didn't care about anything other than health and sperm count. Healthy donor, good swimmers, that's all we wanted. And we got pregnant with his sperm on the first try. Two years later, we got pregnant with his sperm again, also on the first try. In the end, our donor was not Jewish, and we couldn't care less.

Your kids are going to look how they look, and they're going to be interested in what they're interested in, and there is really not much you can do about it. If you're musical and you want your child to be musical, that's great, and you should feel free to look for an egg donor who is musical. But your kid still might not be musical. And if you end up choosing a donor who isn't musically inclined, your kid might be musical anyway just because he or she is raised in your house, where music is important.

At the end of the day, you'll get the child you're meant to have. Nobody ever gets a mini-me of the donor, and two kids from the same donor can turn out completely different. My kids are from the same sperm donor and they are like night and day, with totally different interests and personalities. One is a math/science kid; the other is a theater/humanities kid. And neither is exactly like me, or Natalie, or the donor. This is not cloning. You get what you get, and what you get is what you're meant to have. Trust me, you will adore the child no matter what.

CHAPTER FOUR

Embryos and Conception

IN SOME WAYS, everything up to the point of creating embryos is like the prep work for the marathon. You put all the pieces together, you do your homework and study the course, and now it's race day. Now things are getting real.

Conception is a delicate process—even when a healthy man and a healthy woman are trying to conceive. For successful conception, five things must occur:

1. The woman must ovulate healthy and mature eggs at the appropriate time (when the hormonal environment is conducive to fertilization and pregnancy).

2. The man must ejaculate healthy, mature sperm into or adjacent to the woman's cervix (the passage that links the vagina and the uterus).

3. The physical and chemical environment of the woman's body must promote capacitation (activation) of the sperm as they pass through the reproductive tract toward the egg.

4. The woman must have a healthy fallopian tube that promotes the passage of eggs, sperm, and embryos.

5. The woman must have a healthy uterus, especially the endometrium, with no abnormalities that might hinder implantation and development of an embryo.

Any couple that cannot fulfill all five criteria, for any reason, is unlikely to conceive without assistance.

A Bit of History

In 1944 Dr. John Rock and his assistant Miriam Menkin of Harvard reported that the first US fertilization of human eggs in a laboratory dish (in vitro) had occurred in his lab after six years of trying. They published "In Vitro Fertilization and Cleavage of Human Ovarian Eggs" in the *American Journal of Obstetrics and Gynecology* in 1948. They studied over 800 retrieved eggs and attempted to fertilize 138 of them. Menkin fertilized the eggs from Rock's fertility patients using sperm donated by his medical interns, and then left them to divide, grow, and develop. They even took some of the very first photographs of what they thought were human embryos in the early stages of cell division. The announcement was greeted with interest by the scientific community as well as skepticism, as none of these embryos actually developed into babies. It was later discovered that the cells weren't actually dividing, but were just clumping. But even with this false start Menkin and Rock's research set the wheels in motion for what would be thirty years of IVF research, culminating in the first baby born through IVF in 1978.[1]

Eggs can only be fertilized within a twelve- to twenty-four-hour window, so timing is critical if the sperm are to reach the egg at the proper time. And that is not as easy as it sounds, because the man deposits his sperm in or near the woman's cervix while the egg is several inches away in the fallopian tube, waiting for a healthy and fully capacitated sperm to arrive.

Basically, the sperm propels itself from the cervix to the fallopian tube using its wiggly tail, helped along by peristaltic (wavelike) contractions in the woman's reproductive tract. However, even with the assistance of peristaltic contractions this is not an easy journey for the sperm. Based on relative size, this trip is roughly the same as a full-sized human traveling from Chicago to Honolulu. Unsurprisingly, only a few hundred of the several hundred million sperm the typical man ejaculates survive this twenty-four to forty-eight-hour expedition.

This arduous journey is not without purpose; in fact, it is a vital part of the fertilization process because it facilitates capacitation (activation) of the sperm. Ideally, by the time a sperm reaches the egg, usually about halfway up the fallopian tube, it is fully capacitated, with enzymes housed in the acrosome now freed and available for use in breaking down the zona pellucida (the shell) of the egg.

After fertilization, the egg begins the process of dividing into multiple cells within the zona pellucida, nourished by the ooplasm (the egg white). At the same time, peristaltic contractions push the fertilized egg down the fallopian tube and into the uterus, a process that generally takes three to four days.

A day or two after the fertilized egg reaches the uterus, when it has divided into about a hundred cells, it cracks open and the embryo bursts out. This is known as hatching. Once free of the zona pellucida, the embryo burrows into the endometrium (the lining of the uterus), making contact with the woman's circulatory system and eventually creating a placenta, which provides nutrients and oxygen to the embryo and removes waste products. It is at this stage that the embryo is considered to have successfully implanted and a woman is considered pregnant.

Creating Embryos

As discussed above, five elements are required for successful conception and pregnancy via traditional means. When one or more of these factors can't be met for any reason, the science of assisted reproduction offers viable alternatives. The most common alternatives are in vivo fertilization (fertilization inside the woman's body), in vitro fertilization (fertilization outside the woman's body), and intracytoplasmic sperm injection (a type of in vitro fertilization in which sperm is directly injected into an egg).

In vivo fertilization (AI or IUI). Artificial insemination (or the more politically correct term, alternative insemination) or intrauterine insemination is the simplest way to help a woman conceive. *In vivo* means "in the body." With this process, sperm is inserted into a woman's cervical canal through a catheter, and then nature is left to take its course. This process is relatively simple and risk-free.

In vitro fertilization (IVF). *In vitro* means "outside the body." With this process, sperm and eggs are combined in a petri dish or test tube and fertilization happens outside the woman's body (if all goes well). In vitro fertilization greatly increases the odds of a sperm finding and fertilizing an egg because the distance the sperm needs to travel is significantly reduced.

Intracytoplasmic sperm injection (ICSI). With this process, a single sperm is injected into a retrieved egg using a very thin needle. The embryologist takes care of locating and pene-trating the egg in the petri dish, which means the sperm does not have to do anything except carry healthy chromosomes, thereby ensuring fertilization. If this is the chosen method, all of the retrieved eggs will be fertilized one by one, and with ICSI the fertilization rate is about 70-80%. This can have to do with egg quality, sperm quality, embryologist, equipment and things we do not know.

IVF and ICSI eliminate many of the hurdles that must be overcome with conception. These techniques are especially helpful when a man has inadequate sperm count or poor sperm function, when a woman's reproductive tract is not conducive to fertilization, or when a critical part of the baby-making rec-ipe (sperm or egg) is missing, as with single intended parents and same-sex couples.

Fact: Infertility is not the only reason some women need to use intrauterine insemination (IUI) to get pregnant. Sometimes a woman needs IUI because she experiences pain during intercourse, she's allergic to her partner's sperm, or her partner has an STD so they cannot have sex without a condom.

Cheryl was in her early twenties when she was diagnosed with multiple sclerosis. She and her loving husband, Dean, had always wanted to be parents. However, Cheryl's doctor advised her that carrying a pregnancy could be dangerous and sug-gested she and Dean think about other options. They explored the opportunities available and decided they wanted to have their own biological child. They knew Cheryl couldn't carry a pregnancy, but that didn't mean they couldn't use her eggs and his sperm. And that's just what they did. They created a batch of embryos, and a wonderful surrogate carried and gave birth to a healthy baby for them. Thanks to medical technology and a surrogate, Cheryl and Dean now have the family they always dreamed of.

IVF begins with the creation of a liquid called an insemination medium. The insemination medium both bathes and nourishes the egg (and later the embryo), much as the fluids in a woman's reproductive tract would do. Then sperm are washed in a solution that induces capacitation. Meanwhile, mature eggs are placed in a petri dish containing the insemination medium. When the sperm sample is ready (fully capacitated), a few drops are placed in the petri dish with the eggs and the insemination medium. Then the dish is placed in an incubator and left overnight. Typically, about 70 percent of the eggs will fertilize within a few hours.

Fact: Different doctors create and utilize slightly different insemination mediums, and each doctor is convinced that his or her recipe is the best. However, all insemination mediums are similar in composition. One ingredient is sodium bicarbonate (aka baking soda), which is necessary because eggs and embryos, like all living cells, convert oxygen, food, and water into waste, and they excrete that waste into their surrounding environment. Baking soda neutralizes this waste, just as it neutralizes odors in your refrigerator, safeguarding the well-being of your eggs, sperm, and embryos.

Once created, embryos are kept in an incubator for the next five days. Whatever the embryos need, they get from the insemination medium. They are removed from the incubator during the first five days only to be microscopically examined and graded by the embryologist based on number of cells, symmetry, and overall structure. They are then moved to a fresh medium, frozen, and stored, or are transferred into a womb.

Recently, doctors have begun to use ICSI more often than traditional IVF, primarily because ICSI guarantees fertilization. This process is especially useful if the sperm are not fully motile, because the sperm don't need to swim or travel at all. ICSI bypasses that requirement. All that's needed is sperm with a healthy (chromosomally sound) nucleus.

Are These Technologies Safe?

You might be wondering if all this scientific and medical tinkering will affect the long-term health and well-being of a child. Thankfully, research tells us that it doesn't. A recent study in the medical journal *Fertility and Sterility* found no differences in the physical or mental health of ART adolescents (kids created using assisted reproduction) versus a control group of non-ART adolescents. The research team concluded, "Results provide reassurance that in the long-run health and functioning of ART-conceived adolescents is not compromised."[2] Other studies have found no major differences in birth weight, incidence of birth defects, physical development, overall physical health, IQ, behavior, social development, or any other factor.

Children conceived through assisted reproduction are just as likely to be healthy as non-ART-conceived kids. With multiples (twins, triplets, etc.), there are many health risks that can occur. But these are not the result of the assisted reproductive technologies themselves, but rather the result of higher order pregnancies and the risks that go along with them in any pregnancy.

Embryo Screening

Thanks to consistent improvement in genetic screening techniques, the statement I just made about IVF and ICSI children being just as healthy as other children might actually be an understatement. In time, we may find that children produced via third-party assisted reproduction are somewhat healthier overall than children conceived traditionally because chromosomal screening of embryos, preimplantation, can help us select only those embryos that are likely to result in a healthy child.

I recognize that this is a controversial statement, and I am not weighing in here about the ethics involved. I am just relating the science and the process, and addressing the fears that IVF will introduce health problems in children conceived by this method.

Before chromosomal screening takes place, the embryo is allowed to grow for five or sometimes six days until it reaches the blastocyst (cell differentiation) stage. We often refer to blastocysts as "five-day blasts." Embryos that fail to progress to this stage are always chromosomally abnormal and could never result in a successful pregnancy. So even prior to chromosomal testing doctors can determine which embryos are and are not likely to result in a successful pregnancy.

Not long ago, doctors only waited three days before the embryo transfer to determine the viability of embryos and there was no chromosomal screening. The embryo would grow for three days, the doctor would look at it under a microscope to make sure it looked normal, and then, if it looked okay, the doctor would transfer the embryo and hope for the best. Testing for abnormalities wasn't available until several weeks after the implantation, using amniocentesis. With amniocentesis, at around fourteen to sixteen weeks of pregnancy, the doctor uses a needle to extract some of the amniotic cells and then examines them under a microscope. And this procedure carries some risk to the entire pregnancy.

In the past five years, the science has changed significantly. For starters, we've learned that if we wait until day five or six, the blastocyst stage, we can learn a lot more about the embryo. With blastocysts, preimplantation genetic screening can be performed, greatly increasing the success rate. These tests are optional and your doctor will discuss the risks and benefits, and then you can decide if you want them to be performed.

With PGT-A (preimplantation genetic testing for aneuploidy), the doctor removes five to ten cells from a blastocyst and examines them as thoroughly as possible, checking primarily for chromosomal abnormalities and viability. If the analysis finds problems, that embryo is not selected for transfer. In this way, doctors can cull the abnormal embryos. So, with preimplantation genetic screening intended parents may end up with fewer usable embryos, but they know that the ones they've got are more likely to be healthy and result in a pregnancy.

Genetic screening results take about two weeks and will identify some early chromosomal disorders. Doctors can also see if the cells are doubling and tripling the way they're supposed to. In this way, parents end up with the healthiest embryos and the highest chance that they're going to have a successful pregnancy and a healthy child.

Of course, preimplantation genetic screening is not a guarantee of health. There are some abnormalities that develop and can be detected right from the start, immediately after fertilization, but others start later in the pregnancy. With preimplantation genetic screening we can catch one form but not the other. And there are plenty of things we can't screen for at all, at least not with current technology. For instance, we can't screen for things that occur in later stages of cell division, such as most birth defects, and things for which we haven't identified genetic markers, like autism and depression.

Sex Selection

Preimplantation genetic screening reveals not only potential problems but also the chromosomal sex of the embryo. So you can find out the sex at this point, in addition to the chromosomal quality of the embryo.

Because of this, you can choose the biological sex of your child—though not always, and not with every doctor or in every country. In the United States, even though "sex selection" can be a controversial issue, if you really want a boy or a girl, you can work with a doctor who is willing to let you select which embryo to use. Again, not all doctors will do this; so make sure you ask about this in the beginning if it's important to you.

Fact: We say "sex selection," which has to do with the chromosomes, rather than "gender selection," which is a self-assessment that has to do with society and cultural norms (the way one sees oneself).

Sometimes parents who want twins will choose one of each sex (but not always). Sometimes parents who have one child already will choose a different sex for their second child (but not always). A lot of the time parents don't want to choose, and they leave it up to the doctor. They just want to use the healthiest embryo.

There is no right or wrong approach to sex selection. If you do have a preference, it's important to weigh that with all the other information at hand and communicate ahead of time with your doctor.

How Many Embryos to Transfer

Once embryos have been created and screened, intended parents must decide how many they want to transfer. Generally, if you transfer a single chromosomally healthy embryo, you've got about a 70 percent chance of pregnancy. If you transfer two chromosomally healthy embryos, you've got about a 90 percent chance of pregnancy, with a 50 percent chance of twins. There is also a small chance with multiple embryos that one of the embryos will split and you'll end up with triplets—or even quadruplets, if they both split, but that's very, very rare.

As medical technology changes, these numbers might also change. For now, though, these are the figures. And because the odds of a pregnancy are so high, many doctors recommend single embryo transfers as the best option since pregnancies with multiple babies carry risks. In the past, when IVF procedures were not as good as they are today, doctors would transfer multiple embryos hoping for a single pregnancy. This resulted in several cases of women carrying four or five or more babies when all the embryos took. Still, if transferring single embryos multiple times doesn't work, doctors will transfer more than one embryo to try for a successful pregnancy, as long as everyone is well educated about the risks.

Unfortunately, with twins and triplets the risk for miscarriages and other complications increases dramatically. Triplets are especially risky pregnancies. If you are planning to create and transfer embryos, you have to consider the potential problems that arise with higher order pregnancies. If you choose to transfer twins and something goes wrong, how will you feel about that? And what will you do if one of those eggs splits and suddenly you're looking at triplets?

Bruce and Tammy went back and forth before deciding to transfer two embryos into Tammy, in their third attempt at a pregnancy using their last two embryos. They knew they had only a slight chance of both or even one of the embryos taking, but in their case both embryos implanted. They were thrilled at the positive pregnancy test but then terrified when the ultrasound revealed three heartbeats. They spent a few harrowing weeks figuring out their best course of action, and they finally decided to take a chance and continue with the triplet pregnancy. Tammy ended up on bed rest the last third of her pregnancy and delivered the triplets ten weeks early. The babies stayed in the neonatal intensive care unit (NICU) for several months, until one by one they went home and joined their parents. In this case, the story had a happy ending. But this is not always the case. Triplets are a big risk.

With intended parents going through third-party assisted reproduction or surrogacy, these issues are discussed well in advance, long before it's time to transfer an embryo. Even the surrogate gets a fully informed say, because the more babies she's carrying, the higher her risk is, too. All the options must be placed on the table and fully discussed. Complications and potential action steps are discussed more thoroughly in chapter six.

These days, most intended parents choose to transfer one embryo at a time. If a single embryo is transferred, there is about a 95 percent chance of pregnancy within three tries. Those odds are pretty darn good, so—unless you intentionally want twins—you have a very good chance at success without the risks associated with multiples.

Steve, a single man, wanted twins. He chose to transfer two embryos and his surrogate got pregnant with twins. Sadly, the pregnancy was lost at twenty-two weeks, which is late in the process for a miscarriage, but not completely unheard of—especially with twins. The loss was devastating, and Steve went through quite a bit of grieving. Everything was going great, and then, with no warning or indication that things might not work out, he lost both babies.

For a while, Steve thought he was done, that emotionally he would not be able to try again, even though he had several frozen embryos to work with. He took some time to regroup, got support from his family, friends, and me, and eventually decided to try a single embryo transfer using one of his frozen embryos. The pregnancy was successful, and he had a son. A few years later, Steve came back and used another of his frozen embryos to have a daughter. While the idea of twins was really appealing to him, it just wasn't meant to be. But with time and patience, Steve now has a wonderful family.

Freezing Embryos

Any healthy (chromosomally normal) embryos that are not transferred will be frozen and utilized later if your first attempt does not take, or if you decide you want another child a few years down the road. In fact, both scenarios are common: a couple may transfer from the same batch of embryos two or three times before becoming pregnant, or a couple may have multiple kids from the same batch of embryos, with each of the children gestated in a different pregnancy.

Alan, a single dad, used an egg donor and created a batch of healthy embryos. His doctor transferred one embryo to his surrogate, resulting in his firstborn child—a son. A year later, his doctor transferred two embryos to his surrogate, resulting in his two daughters. Alan likes to joke that his three kids are fraternal triplets that gestated in two batches.

Freezing embryos, technically referred to as cryopreservation, has been around since the 1980s. Back then doctors used a slow freeze process and the survival rate of embryos, on thawing, was around 50 percent. Today we use an ultra-rapid freezing process known as vitrification, which literally freezes cells in the blink of an eye. Vitrification avoids the slow freeze issue of intracellular ice, increasing the post-thaw survival rate to better than 90 percent.

More and more doctors actually prefer to use frozen embryos. As discussed earlier, they can test the embryos for chromosomal health more thoroughly. Plus, when using frozen embryos there is no need to coordinate the reproductive cycles of the egg donor and the intended mother or surrogate, so there is one less factor they need to control. Because there is less coordination involved, using frozen embryos can sometimes speed up the baby-making process. The eggs are harvested when the egg donor is ready, immediately fertilized, and then frozen at the five-day expanded blastocyst stage. After preimplantation testing, the embryos can then be thawed as needed and transferred to the intended mother or surrogate whenever she is ready.

Embryo Donation

At this point you might be wondering, what happens to my embryos when I decide my family is complete? What are my options? The embryos will be stored at the reproductive endocrinologist's office or the lab where they were created. Usually the first year of storage is included in the cost of creating the embryos, and then there will be an annual storage fee somewhere in the neighborhood of $2,000 a year. You could pay for storage indefinitely if you wanted to, but if your family is complete and you know you will never use them, you can have the remaining embryos destroyed by the embryologist. Depending on the country's political environment and the current status of stem cell research, you could alternatively donate the embryos to science. You can also donate your healthy embryos to another couple so that they can have a baby.

There are no right or wrong answers here. Each person has a unique set of values and core beliefs that will influence his or her decision. That said, I think it's awesome when people decide to donate their unused embryos to people who want to be parents but can't seem to make it happen with their own embryos, no matter how hard they try.

Not everyone is willing to do this, of course, because any children born using donated embryos will be genetically related to the parents' own kids. So before donating they must ask themselves, "How will I feel about this? Will I feel proud, ashamed, confused, worried? How will I explain this scenario to my children?" Plenty of parents are fine with donating their unused embryos, and an agency should help facilitate this donation. There should not be any fees for this. In fact, embryo recipients cannot legally pay for embryos; there will be some legal and medical fees, but no payment for the embryos. It's a donation and should be treated as such, start to finish. There are legal contracts that protect this process, but these are straightforward.

We sometimes have clients who've had their children, and they know without a doubt that they don't want more. Still, they don't want to destroy their embryos, and they'll ask if we know anyone who might want their unused embryos. Meanwhile, we've got another couple that has been totally out of luck in their attempts to build their family. They are in that 1 percent of people who've gone through a bunch of embryo transfers with multiple egg donors or multiple surrogates and nothing has worked. They're tapped out financially and they're emotionally beaten, but they don't want to give up. Through the generosity of those people willing to donate their embryos, we're often able to make these people's dreams of parenthood come true.

Fact: Most of the time an agency will not ask people if they want to donate their embryos—parents just indicate that they are willing, and then, before you know it, a couple in need suddenly appears. It's absolutely amazing. And, once again, people end up with the baby they're meant to have.

Through egg donation and IVF, Gregg and Edgar ended up with twelve frozen embryos. They transferred one to their surrogate, who became pregnant with their first daughter. Two years later they had a son with the help of another surrogate. About a year after that, they called me asking for advice about what to do with their remaining embryos. They knew they were done having kids and wanted to help someone else in the way that their donor and surrogates had helped them. They asked me if we ever have intended parents who have financial hardship and could use the help. I told them I would keep an eye out. The next month, Tom and Elaine, a couple that had been struggling with infertility for years and could not produce embryos of their own, were about to give up. I connected the two families through a fertility attorney who helped facilitate the embryo donation. Tom and Elaine had a set of twins with the help of a surrogate and forever consider Gregg and Edgar (whom they never met) their extended family for giving them such a precious gift.

One potentially complicating factor with embryo donation is that the egg donor has legally donated to one couple but not the other. A good agency will discuss the possibility of embryo donation with egg donors up front, and most donors are totally fine with the idea. In the case above, the egg donor had agreed in advance that Gregg and Edgar could donate or dispose of their embryos as they saw fit.

As with every aspect of assisted reproduction, embryo donation is a process that everyone needs to be completely open and honest about. Sometimes it is done anonymously, like Gregg and Edgar did with Tom and Elaine, and sometimes it's done openly and the two families end up as friends, getting to know each other, staying in touch, and watching each other's families grow. Whatever the preference and whatever the process, embryo donation is a very generous act.

CHAPTER FIVE

The Womb and Surrogacy

EVERY HUMAN BEING has its beginnings in the same place: a woman's womb. Nourished and protected, the growing fetus spends approximately forty weeks gestating until it's big enough to join its parents. This part of the ART marathon is thrilling, exciting, and terrifying, yet filled with hope and anticipation.

When the Intended Mother Provides the Womb

Sometimes an intended mother is perfectly capable of carrying a healthy baby to term but she can't produce an egg or an embryo. In such cases, an embryo can be created using an egg donor, and then transferred into the mother.

Some intended parents have strong feelings about using an embryo to which they did not genetically contribute. They might wonder, "Who is this baby going to be? Will this baby really be my child?" If you find yourself feeling this way, rest assured that your baby will truly be yours, and you will bond with it just like any other parent and child when the time comes.

That time might be when the embryo is created, it might be at transfer or confirmation of pregnancy, it might be the first ultrasound that shows a heartbeat, it might be at birth, or it might be when your baby comes home. But it *will* happen.

This variation in the timing and style of bonding occurs not just with assisted reproduction but also with parenthood in general. Mothers and fathers bond at different times and in different ways. Sometimes intended mothers who carry an embryo created with the help of an egg donor attribute their lack of early bonding to using another woman's egg, but that's really not the defining factor. In reality, some women don't bond early or at all during the pregnancy. Instead, they bond after birth or while nursing (if they choose to nurse). Many parents do bond with their unborn baby, but just as many do not, and this is true whether you build your family with the help of assisted reproduction or not.[1] So if you are worried because you are not bonding with your unborn child—whether you are carrying it or a surrogate is carrying it, rest assured your feelings and process are normal.

When the Surrogate Provides the Womb

Again, all babies develop in a womb. If you don't have one or medical problems exist, you will need the help of a gestational surrogate to grow your baby. Gestational surrogates are women who provide a "host" womb, carrying and giving birth to another person's baby. They do not genetically contribute to the baby. (Historically, some women were traditional surrogates, women who become pregnant through insemination rather than IVF, but this is not very popular anymore and rarely done.)

Surrogates are usually paid between $25,000 and $35,000. They are paid throughout the process with larger payments at various milestones (like when they start injections or hit a marker in the pregnancy). Then they are paid the balance of the fee after the baby is born. The range of fees has to do with various factors. For example, if a surrogate is carrying twins, she is better compensated for the increased wear and tear on her body. If she is an experienced surrogate, she will also be paid a bit more. All of this will be spelled out in the contract. However, women do not become surrogates for the money. Frankly, there is not enough money in the world to properly compensate them. After all, they must endure screenings and shots and medications and all sorts of minor and occasionally major inconveniences. They hear things like, "You have to be at the doctor's office tomorrow morning at nine, and I'm sorry that it's your daughter's turn for show and tell and you're going to have to miss it." Or sometimes they hear much worse, like, "You'll need full bed rest for the next eight weeks, which means you can't go to work or help around the house or attend your child's school play and ballgames."

So why, you might ask, would any woman put herself through this intense process? There is a very good answer to that question. She does it because she is one of the nicest and most generous people on earth.

Often these women are either stay-at-home supermoms or they're in a helping profession. A lot of them are nurses, teachers, or childcare providers who *love* what they do. The desire to be of service is a dominant personality trait of all surrogates. They are incredibly caring, bighearted women. They help people whenever they can, no matter the inconvenience. They donate blood, they volunteer at the local soup kitchen, and they would donate a kidney if someone needed it. If they had an extra $100,000, they would give it to charity. In short, surrogates want to make the world a better place, and they're willing to sacrifice in all sorts of amazing ways to make that happen.[2]

Surrogate Kelly has given birth to eight babies—three of her own and five for other families. Not long ago, one of Kelly's own kids, her nine-year-old son Sawyer, passed away of lymphoma. Since Kelly is a frequent and well-known blogger about surrogacy and related topics, she was able to share openly with other surrogates about Sawyer's illness and his passing. I watched as the community of surrogates walked this tragic journey with Kelly, banding together, sharing her grief, and raising money to help with medical bills and other expenses. They wept with her and for her. I have never, not even once, seen or felt this degree of empathy in any other community. But I witness this level of love from surrogates 24/7/365.

Interestingly, surrogates don't see themselves as making a baby. They know that the intended parents are making the baby. They are making a family. They don't think of the baby as their own, so when the baby is born they are not giving it up; they're giving it back. That is a very important distinction. The baby belongs to the parents, not the surrogate. One of the most poignant moments for the surrogate is when the parents see their baby for the first time. That one moment is the ultimate payoff for a surrogate. The joy they experience from giving people a gift that they can't otherwise receive is what motivates them to do what they do.

You might remember Alan from the previous chapter, the single man with fraternal triplets gestated in two batches. I'll never forget his mother taking me in her arms after the first child was born and thanking me for making her a grandma. While I wasn't their surrogate, that experience is gold for me, and that is why I do what I do.

Not long ago, a surrogate sent me an essay that her nine-year-old daughter wrote for school. This woman is a home daycare provider, and her daughter's essay was about her hero. The little girl wrote, in part, "My mother is my hero because she takes care of other people's babies, sometimes in our house, and sometimes in her body." I think that pretty much says it all.

Screening Potential Surrogates

A good agency will conduct a comprehensive screening of potential surrogates. That said, there are a few basic requirements that should be met before a woman is even considered as a potential candidate. First and foremost, she must already be a mother. She must have given birth at least once, to her own child or children. Moreover, her family must be complete, or at least she must feel okay about not having more kids of her own. This is primarily because pregnancies and births are risky, and surrogacy could damage a woman's ability to have more babies of her own.

Surrogates should also have a certain minimum income level. They can't be on welfare, state aid, food stamps, or other kinds of aid. A reputable agency will make sure potential surrogates are not doing it for the money, so they won't ever feel exploited. If a woman became a surrogate because she was desperate for money, we'd be taking advantage of her, and we'd also get candidates who aren't as likely to do all the things that surrogates must do while pregnant, like eating right and making all the scheduled doctor's visits. With ethical surrogacy, it's very important that surrogates not "rent their wombs" as a way to pay the bills. Instead, we're looking for women who know the joys of motherhood and want to help others become parents in a beautiful and intentional collaboration.

Surrogates must also be generally healthy. They don't have to be super fit, but they do have to be within certain BMI (body mass index) parameters, because the doctors we work with all require that. This requirement is based on looking after the overall well-being of the surrogate and the baby.

Surrogates also need social and familial support from others for what they're doing. If they're in a long-term relationship, their husband or partner needs to completely accept their choice to be a surrogate, because it is definitely a team effort. If they're single, they need to have the support of relatives, close friends, and the like. Carrying and delivering a baby is not easy, and like any pregnant woman, they will experience emotional ups and downs, they will need help with all sorts of everyday tasks, and they will need care when they don't feel well. If they don't have good support at home and from their friends, life can get really difficult, really quickly. It's important to ensure they're not in this alone.

Surrogates must also live in a state where surrogacy is legally sanctioned, where the surrogacy contract will be upheld based on state laws and precedent. This is to protect and ensure the rights of the intended parents. As of this writing, there are about thirty states where surrogacy is legal, where the legal rights of the intended parents, including the right to make medical decisions concerning the health of their unborn child, are paramount. In addition, each state in the United States has a different way of establishing the parental rights after the baby is born. Some states, through what is called a pre-birth judgment, put the parents'—and only the parents'—names on the birth certificate. Other states require a court order after birth to amend a birth certificate. Some states even require the parents to adopt their baby. In some states both parents must be genetically related to the child to be on the birth certificate. So it is important that your surrogate lives in a state where your parental rights can be established and that you know what that process will be before you get started. Your agency or attorney will know which states will work for you based on your family type (heterosexual, gay or lesbian, married, not married), whether or not you are using your own genetics or donor genetics, and your country of origin requirements if you are not in the United States.

Most agencies require that surrogates live near a high-level neonatal intensive care unit (NICU) in case there are complications with the baby or delivery. This requirement adds a level of assurance that should a problem or complication arise, the surrogate will have access to expert care. It also means your surrogate won't deliver your baby in a rural doctor's office or a small hospital that's not equipped to handle major problems.

Scott and Shauna's surrogate, Trina, was twenty-five weeks pregnant with twins when she started having what she thought were contractions. Trina immediately went to the ER/NICU, and it was determined that her cervix was beginning to open, a dangerous situation that could lead to early delivery. Because Trina knew what signs to look for and acted quickly, her doctor was able to perform a procedure called a cerclage, which is a method of stitching the cervix closed and temporarily preventing delivery, averting what could have been a tragedy. Because of Trina's quick response and the expertise of some highly trained medical personnel, she was able to carry the twins to full term. The cerclage was removed at thirty-five weeks, and Trina went into labor naturally about a week later and delivered two healthy babies into the waiting arms of Scott and Shauna.

If a potential surrogate meets all the above criteria, a second level of screening should be conducted, which is incredibly in depth. For starters, there is a criminal background check of not only the surrogate but also her spouse if she's married. The potential surrogate's driving records and taxes are reviewed. If those records are clean, lengthy interviews are held with the candidate and her main emotional support—her spouse, her mom, her best friend, and anyone else who will be a key ally during the process. And if things are still looking good, a mental health professional conducts an in-person psychological evaluation, and a reproductive endocrinologist orders an array of medical tests, including a head-to-toe physical, blood work, and a uterine ultrasound. Start to finish, the screening process takes around six months.

Fact: In my practice, fewer than three out of one hundred women who apply to be a surrogate make it all the way through the screening. Surrogates are the keystones of this process, and rigorous screening tells us if they're a good fit for surrogacy before proceeding.

Being a surrogate can be hugely inconvenient. The women who get this far have been pregnant before, so they know that pregnancy is not easy, but we remind them. Generally, they are accomplished people with a lot on their plates. Even if they're stay-at-home moms, they're in charge of the soccer league or president of the PTA. If a surrogate needs bed rest or she misses work due to the pregnancy, she is compensated, and will also have an allowance for childcare and housekeeping if she needs it—these costs should be included in the total benefit package outlined in the contract. But even with the support and compensation, it is a lot to expect a surrogate to be stuck in bed for a day, or a week, or even a couple of months. A good agency will want to make sure she is absolutely ready for that, and will want to assess how she'll cope in this kind of circumstance. I know what it's like when I'm at home sick. Day one is great. I sleep a lot and maybe catch up on my shows. Day two is more of the same, but maybe less sleep and more TV. Day three, I really want to get out of bed. I have to remind surrogates that things like this might happen, and if they do, they'll have to deal with it.

The goal, in addition to making sure your surrogate wants to be a surrogate for all the right reasons, is to minimize surprises. Surrogacy can be incredibly inconvenient, and as with any pregnancy, almost nothing happens on a preferred timeline—and it's important to be prepared for that. So making sure that the surrogate is on board for the level of flexibility required is very important.

For example, let's say an embryo transfer is scheduled for Friday. Your surrogate will be flying in on Thursday and spending Thursday night in a hotel. (Side note: Most matches are not necessarily nearby. We'll discuss this more later on.) The embryo transfer will happen on Friday. Saturday she'll rest, and Sunday she'll catch a flight home. Monday she'll be back at work, with three important meetings, and that night she'll be leading the meeting for her daughter's Girl Scout troop. The schedule should work, right? But then the doctor decides the embryos need another twenty-four hours to grow, and the transfer gets pushed back a day. Now your surrogate won't be home on Monday, her whole schedule is messed up, and there's nothing that can really be done about it. You want to make sure in advance that she is prepared for situations like these. Because they are bound to happen.

Surrogates are not putting their entire lives on hold, but there are definitely days when they have to put surrogacy first. Usually, they can count on at least a month of serious inconvenience. Those days typically don't happen all together, thankfully, but they do happen and it can be difficult to manage. It's imperative that your surrogate can deal with the inconveniences.

Fact: Women who've already been a surrogate must be rescreened if they want to be a surrogate again. Despite the time and expense involved, it's important to be certain that no medical issues or other developments have come up in the interim.

You can't be overly cautious when you're screening a potential surrogate, and I'll give you a real-world example why. A gay couple decided to use the sister of one of the men as their surrogate. She lived in a state that does not legally support the intended parents in a surrogacy arrangement. This factor alone should have disqualified her from being a surrogate, but this couple did not work with an agency, or hire an attorney, so they didn't realize the laws that would affect their situation, nor did they conduct a psychological screening on the sister.

One of the men gave sperm, which was used to inseminate a batch of eggs from a donor. Two of those eggs were selected and implanted in the surrogate. She got pregnant with twins, two girls, and gave birth to them in her home state, where surrogacy is not legally protected. Then the sister decided she wanted to keep the babies as her own. Because she lived in and gave birth to the babies in a state without protection for the intended parents, the courts protected her instead of the intended parents. The kids are about ten years old now, and to this day the fathers do not have custody.

This sad situation could have been avoided. The surrogate, simply by living where she did, should not have been a surrogate. If there were legal documents in place clearly stating everyone's intent, they would have protected the intended parents. And without doubt, a psychological screening would have eliminated the sister as an appropriate candidate had that evaluation ever been performed. But none of those precautions were taken.

Just because your sister volunteers to be your surrogate doesn't mean you don't need to take the same precautions you would take with an unknown candidate. You may love each other, but a lot can go wrong. As the saying goes, you don't know what you don't know; and engaging the services of professionals can go a long way to help you anticipate problems and make a plan for how to handle those problems should they arise. This is what we call ethical surrogacy. These steps should not be skipped. Not ever. Not for any reason.

Are Parents Screened?

Intended parents are also screened. For starters, there will be a criminal background check and a thorough medical screening. Most medical issues will not preclude an intended parent from having a baby with a surrogate, but it's important to make sure everyone is fully informed about any issues they may need to deal with in addition to becoming a parent. Some kind of psycho-educational consultation will also occur. This is to make sure the intended parent is fully informed about the psychological and emotional rigors of third-party assisted reproduction, and is also an opportunity to ask any questions that remain.

There are a couple of reasons intended parents may be turned away. If the potential intended parent fails the background check, they may not be able to be matched with a surrogate. Minor issues are not a problem. For instance, if a couple in their mid-thirties wants to have a baby and one of them had a DUI or passed a bad check in college, with nothing since, that's probably okay. But more serious issues could get in the way—especially if there was any aggressive or dangerous behavior in the past. A surrogate will not likely want to carry a baby for someone who committed a violent crime, for example, for obvious reasons.

Another issue that may interfere with surrogacy is when the potential intended parent insists on withholding information or keeping secrets from the surrogate. For instance, my agency turned down a wonderful couple that came to see us because the wife could not bear children. She was transgender, born male but now female, so she didn't have a uterus. The couple did not want to share this information with the surrogate. Reluctantly, we turned them down. We were happy to work with a transgender woman, but we were not willing to hide that information from the surrogate. We easily could have located a willing egg donor and surrogate, but the couple refused to be fully open. A cornerstone of ethical third-party assisted reproduction is that everyone is fully informed at all times. Trust and truth are necessary foundations.

One parental screening I did several years ago reveals the importance of truth in this process. Tim and Maggie were a slightly older couple—Maggie was in her late forties and Tim was in his early sixties. Tim already had grown kids from a previous marriage and Maggie wanted to have one of her own via surrogacy. But there was a medical complication: Tim had cancer. The illness was in remission, but there was a good chance it might return. During our initial consultation, Maggie left the room at one point to go to the restroom. Tim took my hand and said in a low, serious voice, "I bet you wonder why I'm doing this, why I want to start all over with a baby when I already have children and my own health is in question. Well, I love Maggie, and if I were not around for a long time with her, I would be honored to leave a piece of myself with her. I'm doing this for her and for us."

We agreed to help Tim and Maggie with no reservations whatsoever. Life is uncertain, sometimes more so than others, but that's not a reason to stop living. A few months after Tim and Maggie's son was born, Tim's cancer returned, and within two years he was gone. But his memory, the love he had for Maggie, and his gorgeous son remain.

Some professionals won't work with heterosexual couples who are fertile but don't want to carry the baby. Their argument is that pregnancy carries a risk, and that risk should not be transferred to someone else simply because the wife doesn't want to carry the baby or give birth. That same argument could be used against helping gay men become parents, as there are children available for adoption, and they could become parents without introducing risk to someone else. Adoption is wonderful, but it's not for everyone—and it's not always available to everyone. The same is true with third-party assisted reproduction. I will work with anyone as long as they are fully transparent up front. If all parties are screened, informed, educated, and consenting, the process is ethical.

Using a Known Surrogate

A known surrogate is a woman you know before the surrogacy process begins. Usually, a known surrogate is a sister, cousin, or close friend of an intended parent. An unknown surrogate is a woman you don't know before the process starts. By the end, obviously, you will know her very well; but she was not in your life before the surrogacy, and her role in your life is to be the surrogate carrying your child.

In many ways, issues related to using a known versus an unknown surrogate are the same as with known versus anonymous sperm and egg donors. However, in a few ways the situation with surrogates is slightly less fraught, because a known surrogate is not genetically connected to your child or children, whereas a sperm and egg donor are. But it's still a highly charged experience, with all sorts of issues to consider. And all of those possibilities must absolutely be discussed up front.

If you plan to use your sister or your best gal pal as your surrogate, she's going to be in your life, and she's going to be around any of your children that she carries and gives birth to. So you need to ask yourself the following questions before moving forward:

- How will you feel about your surrogate being around your children as they grow up?

- How will she feel about being around your child that she gave birth to?

- Will she be able to feel like the aunt and not the mom, even after she gives birth?

- What if she doesn't pass the screening because things don't check out either psychologically or medically? How will you feel about that? How will she feel about that?

- What if she does pass the screening and you move forward but something goes horribly wrong with the process? What if your baby does not make it? What if she loses her uterus because of complications with the pregnancy and/or the birth?

- Will one or both of you forever feel guilty?

Another issue to consider is that if you use a sibling, cousin, or close friend as your surrogate, you are taking her out of your support network as related to the surrogacy process. In other words, a person you might normally rely on in difficult moments is no longer fully available to support you. In fact, you may end up needing to support her during the rough patches. Are you okay with that? Is she okay with that? And, just as importantly, is your support network strong enough that you're willing to remove a key element of it?

In cases where intended parents come to me with a potential surrogate in mind, I always ask the same question: Whose idea was it for her to carry your baby? With a surrogate provided through an agency, the idea was the surrogate's. She came to surrogacy because she wanted to do this. With a known surrogate, that's not always the case. If your sister comes to you and says, "Gosh, I think you'd be great parents, and I know you really want this. I'd be honored to carry your baby for you," that's one thing. But if you approached her, that's another thing entirely. She might feel obligated or pressured to help, or as if she couldn't bear to let you down. An initially unknown surrogate's motivation is helping you create a family; your sister's motivations might be very different.

There are a lot of considerations if you want to use a known surrogate, which is probably why the vast majority of intended parents opt for a surrogate met through an agency. But with lots of preplanning and conversations, either option can work.

Finding the Right Surrogate for You

Unlike sperm and egg donation, which are at the complete discretion of the intended parents, surrogacy is a mutual arrangement.

Not every surrogate who passes the screening is right for every intended parent. Because the screenings are so thorough, all fully screened surrogates are wonderful, but the goal is to facilitate the best possible match, taking all factors into account. Factors to consider include demographic issues that matter to the intended parents (such as the surrogate's marital status, where she lives, or her employment status), along with the surrogate's wants and needs. Sometimes a surrogate really wants to work with a gay couple because she knows that's the only way those men can have a baby. Other times a surrogate is fine with the idea of helping a gay couple but her church or family would not support it. In these cases, the surrogate should help a heterosexual couple or a straight single person.

Sometimes intended parents want the surrogate to be nearby so they can stay in closer physical contact. Other times they'd prefer a bit of distance. In all cases there is plenty of interaction, and the expectations of both intended parents and the surrogate need to be aligned. Otherwise, they're going to get on each other's nerves—and this process is hard enough without that extra level of tension. It's also important to consider your style of relating. For example, some people are warm and fuzzy and big on hugs. Others, not so much. It's important to match surrogates and parents who feel the same way about these sorts of things. The bottom line is that no matter what kind of relationship the surrogate and parents are having, they need to be on the same page. So the parameters, the expectations, the wants and needs of that relationship need to be expressed in the beginning.

Surrogacy is, after all, a collaboration of fully informed consenting adults coming together with one goal: to help create a family. And at the center of that collaboration are the surrogate and the intended parents. As with any collaboration, the things that make it work are trust, communication, flexibility, honesty, mutual respect, and partnership.

Most agencies pair intended parents and surrogates in a similar fashion. When they think they have a match, they'll send the intended parents' profile to the surrogate first. She looks it over, and then she says yes or no to that profile. If she says yes, the agency will send the surrogate's profile to the intended parents. If they also like what they see on paper, a match meeting will be set up.

At the first match meeting, a counselor reviews everything that's involved in the parent-surrogate relationship: how each party likes to communicate, how often they want to communicate, who will attend doctor's visits, how medical care will be provided, who will be in the delivery room. They also discuss a whole host of possible complications that might arise and what all parties will do if one of these situations happens. What will the parents do if something is found to be wrong with the developing fetus? Would the surrogate agree to let the parents make the choice to continue or terminate the pregnancy? What if there are multiples? Is the surrogate willing to carry multiple children? Diet and setting personal boundaries are also discussed. After the baby is born, do the parents want the surrogate to pump breast milk for the baby? And is she willing to do that?

After the surrogate and intended parents meet, there is a short waiting period before either party decides. These meetings can be exciting, and it can be easy to get caught up in the euphoria of the moment. That's why it's important to take some time to carefully consider all aspects of the relationship, including possible conflicts.

When this degree of attention and care to matching is followed, almost all of the suggested matches are confirmed. The parents and the surrogate like each other, they feel good about the pairing, and they want to move forward. Once in a while, for whatever reason, someone says no. A rejected match is not the end of the world. It just means the agency will look for a better match, and when they think they've found one, they will try again. As my grandmother used to say, not every lid fits every pot, but every pot has a lid that fits.

With matchmaking, you're not looking for a new best friend; you're looking for a woman you can trust and communicate with. Do you trust her to carry and give birth to your baby? Can you communicate effectively with her, and she with you? That's what you're looking for. Still, plenty of parents and surrogates develop lasting friendships—everything from sending annual holiday cards to becoming extended family and going on vacations together. But that type of close bond is not a prerequisite for successful surrogacy. Trust and communication are much more important.

My favorite match story is not really about the match, but about two couples that met at a party one night. They got to talking and realized they'd each had boy-girl twins via surrogacy. They started swapping stories, including talk about how much each couple loved their surrogate. One couple mentioned how they'd even gone to see their surrogate, Vickye, in Oregon, where she lives, and the other couple gasped. They'd used the same surrogate! The two families quickly became great friends, and now they are an extended family. The matches we made for two different couples and the same surrogate were so good that the couples and their kids were a match, too.

Later, when Vickye heard about this, she told me, "Finding out they know each other, two families in a city of millions, was incredible. I just find it amazing that I helped create two different families, and then they found each other completely by accident and became great friends. That just confirms for me that this was all meant to be."

The Surrogate's Role

The surrogate's primary role is to be a healthy pregnant person, and to allow the intended parents to be parents even while she's pregnant, sharing important moments and feeling joyful. Beyond that, it's a matter of ongoing communication, which is why the right match is so important. If the surrogate's style and the client's style are well matched, effective communication occurs relatively easily, even during the inevitable difficult moments.

Earlier in this chapter I introduced Kelly, who's given birth to three children of her own and five children for three other families. As mentioned, she is a frequent blogger. One of my favorite postings of hers, on why she loves being a surrogate and how she views her role, reads as follows:

I am a mother and then some.

Since 2001, I have given birth to eight healthy babies. I don't actually have eight kids running around my house, but eight healthy embryos have flourished in my uterus over the years. Three of those were my own children and the other five grew into babies for three other families. You see, I am not just a mother, I am a gestational surrogate. And even though I'm not the mother of my surrogate babies with every hope their parents had, every pregnancy, every birth, every experience of placing a newborn in its parent's arms caused me to relive my own journey to motherhood. As I helped others realize their dreams of becoming parents, I was continually reminded how truly amazing being a mother can be. It takes a very special mom to become a surrogate. For only mothers truly understand the gift they are giving and the amazing lessons of love and family their own children are about to learn. These surrogates are teachers, nurses, day care providers, etc., but above all, they are mothers. I will always be a mother. It's part of who I am. And I will always be a surrogate. It, too, is part of who I am. Years from now I will look back at my experiences and I will swell with pride when I think of the families I helped create. Not just my own, but six other parents who have been able to live the dream. Yes, I am a mother, and then some.

CHAPTER SIX

Pregnancy and Birth

PREGNANCY IS A MAJOR MILESTONE on the marathon of assisted reproduction. For many intended parents, the embryo transfer is the very last step before the wait for the pregnancy test and the hopeful, happy news; but a positive pregnancy test will often be met with disbelief and even mistrust given what intended parents have been through to get to this point. It can be very hard to believe that things will work out. So finally achieving a pregnancy is a milestone, but there's still quite a bit of the race still ahead.

The Basic Science of the Embryo Transfer

The embryo transfer, the procedure where the fertilized embryos are placed inside the uterus, is an exciting event. If the doctor likes to transfer fresh embryos, he or she will have coordinated the reproductive cycles of the egg donor and the intended mother or surrogate, ensuring the carrier's reproductive tract is primed for successful transfer five days after the eggs are harvested and fertilized. If the doctor prefers working with frozen embryos (the growing trend), the prep work is the same except the reproductive cycles of the egg donor and the intended mother or surrogate need not be synchronized.

To prepare the carrier's womb for the embryo transfer and pregnancy (and, if desired, to control the timing of her reproductive cycle), she is given estradiol in the form of injections, pills, or patches, with regular blood tests measuring her levels so the doctor can determine the subsequent dosage. This goes on for four to six weeks, or maybe a bit longer if necessary. There are lots of medications to keep track of at this point in the process, which is not a lot of fun for anyone—but remembering the end goal helps a lot. After the second week of these medications the doctor examines the carrier's uterus via ultrasound to evaluate the development of the endometrium, the uterine lining. When the doctor feels comfortable that the lining is progressing and thickening as hoped and the hormone levels are appropriate, the embryo transfer is scheduled. Several days before the transfer, the carrier receives daily injections of progesterone to optimize endometrial readiness.

The actual embryo transfer procedure sounds simple and straightforward, but it is actually quite delicate. When the intended mother is going to be the carrier, her husband or partner is usually with her for the embryo transfer. When the surrogate is the carrier, she also brings at least one person to support her. This might be her husband or her partner, or it might be her mom, her sister, or a close friend. Often the intended parents are also present, though sometimes they aren't. It depends on what they want and what the surrogate and the doctor are comfortable with. But most of the time the intended parents want to be there, and everybody is fine with that arrangement. With many reproductive endocrinologists, if the intended parents can't be there in person they can watch through a video link.

The embryos are prepared for the transfer by the embryologist affiliated with the fertility doctor, often at the same site, and are brought into the room in an incubator and ready for insertion. Typically, the intended parents can view the embryos via microscope, or microscopic images of the embryos are flashed on a screen for everyone to see. The embryos look nothing like a baby at this point, but like a bunch of little circles stuck together in a lump. It's exciting nonetheless.

Most doctors want the intended mother or the surrogate to be in a relaxed state for the embryo transfer, primarily because certain hormones and neurotransmitters (like adrenaline) are released during stressful events, and these may cause the uterus to contract, thereby making implantation more difficult. To achieve a more peaceful state, some doctors use breathing techniques and/or visualization techniques. Others administer a small dose of valium (or a similar medication) shortly before the procedure.

Fact: Embryo transfers work best when the intended carrier has a full bladder. This doesn't help with tension and anxiety, but it does facilitate ultrasound imagery of the uterus. It also triggers a reflex response that relaxes the endometrium, significantly reducing the potential for muscular contractions that might expel a recently implanted embryo.

An embryo transfer is not a surgical procedure in the traditional sense, and there is no need for anesthesia. The doctor inserts a speculum into the woman's vagina to expose the cervix. Then, an abdominal ultrasound transducer is placed on the woman's lower abdomen. At that point, the woman's reproductive system is clearly visible to the doctor on a video screen.

With video assistance, the doctor gently places a catheter through the woman's vagina, past her cervix, and into the uterine cavity. When the catheter is in place, the doctor injects an embryo into the uterus. If twins are desired, two embryos are injected at the same time. Generally, the depth of the woman's uterus has been measured on a previous ultrasound and the doctor has chosen a specific spot, usually near the top of the uterus, for the placement of the embryo. After the embryo(s) are released inside the uterus, the catheter is slowly withdrawn.

The entire procedure takes five minutes at most. Immediately afterward, the woman may or may not feel some minor lower abdominal pain. She might also have a slight discharge. Both responses are perfectly normal, and neither is problematic.

Some doctors require that a woman rest after the procedure. This rest is probably unnecessary, given the fact that people get pregnant when they go dancing, sneak off to the coatroom to have sex, and then immediately dance and party for another five hours. However, because this process is so intentional, resting for an hour or two afterward can't hurt. Her support person keeps her company. The intended parents can do that as well, if that's what the surrogate and the parents decide they want.

After the woman is released, she usually takes it easy for another day or two, returning to light to normal activity, just to give the embryo(s) the best chance to latch on. Once again, this is probably unnecessary, but most women choose to do this. After a couple of days, however, it's business as usual—back to work, parenting, and all the other things women do on a normal day.

Pregnancy

A woman is considered pregnant when a fertilized embryo has implanted into the uterine wall. This can take between one and five days after the embryo transfer. There are two types of pregnancy, and it's important to note the difference. A chemical pregnancy is when a blood or urine test confirms a pregnancy. These tests tell us that there is an embryo secreting pregnancy hormones into the woman's body. Chemical pregnancy can be detected about seven days after implantation. Clinical pregnancy, when pregnancy is visually confirmed by an ultrasound showing a healthy fetus with a heartbeat, can't be confirmed for another six weeks, give or take.

When a clinical pregnancy is confirmed, there is an 85 percent (or better) chance that the pregnancy will proceed normally and a healthy baby will be born. If things still look good at the twelve-week mark, the odds increase to around 95 percent.

Prior to the six-week mark there is a lot that can go wrong. For instance, the embryo may not implant properly, or the embryo might not be as chromosomally viable as originally thought when it was first examined and tested. There will also be some pregnancies that just don't take and we'll never know why.

With IVF, about 20 percent of chemical pregnancies are lost before they are clinically confirmed. Most likely this is the same rate as with any pregnancy, though we don't know for sure because most women don't even think about a urine or blood pregnancy test until they're at least a few weeks late with their period (i.e., at around the six-week mark). With assisted reproduction, the statistics are available because the chemical pregnancy is confirmed shortly after implantation.

Many women who are not intentionally trying to get pregnant and have had an early miscarriage typically don't even know that it's happened. If a woman has sex, gets pregnant, and prior to the six-week mark something goes wrong with the pregnancy, she'll have a heavy and unpleasant period. But unless she's either very in tune with her body or has been tracking her fertility, she may not recognize that as evidence of a miscarriage. With assisted reproduction, since the doctor is closely monitoring the process, pregnancy can be confirmed early on, so a loss is definitely recognized.

Because early miscarriages happen so often, it's important to realize that a pregnancy is not a clinical pregnancy until it's confirmed with an ultrasound, six weeks after the embryo transfer. Still, it's difficult to not be excited when the chemical pregnancy test is positive, as it is a huge milestone in the marathon of assisted reproduction, and it is often the first time hopeful intended parents have received good news.

I actually had an early miscarriage before I had my first child. But the only reason I knew about it was Natalie and I were trying to get pregnant and we'd detected a chemical pregnancy after one of the insemination attempts. The experience wasn't all that traumatic for me because I understood the process, but I remember it to this day. I remember where I was the moment I knew, what I thought, what I felt, all of it. It was a very emotional experience, but it didn't destroy me, and it didn't make me think I wouldn't eventually become a mother. It was a very difficult experience, but I understood that it was part of the process, and I was committed to trying again.

Fact: Early miscarriages are often nature's way of taking care of the family, recognizing that the embryo was not going to develop into a healthy baby. Either the carrier's body sensed that something was seriously wrong, or the embryo sloughed off on its own because it wasn't able to latch on and develop in a healthy way.

After the embryo transfer, the intended mother or surrogate typically receives daily progesterone injections and biweekly estrogen injections, pills, or patches to sustain an optimal uterine environment. Ten days to two weeks after the embryo transfer, she is tested for chemical pregnancy. A positive test suggests implantation is taking place. If chemical pregnancy is detected, the hormone injections continue for another four to six weeks. If not, the hormone treatments are discontinued, and the woman will typically menstruate within three to ten days.

If the test for chemical pregnancy is positive, of course everybody is very happy; but, as mentioned earlier, we try to temper expectations until a clinical pregnancy is confirmed via ultrasound. If everything looks good on the six weeks ultrasound, we do another at eight or nine weeks, along with multiple blood tests. If things still look fine, the reproductive endocrinologist will release the newly pregnant woman to her obstetrician in ten to twelve weeks.

The first doctor, the reproductive endocrinologist, is there for all the prep work, the embryo transfer, and the first trimester, running that leg of the marathon with the parents. Then an obstetrician will take over her care. If the woman has a long history of infertility, there may be more scrutiny of her pregnancy; but once the pregnancy is well established, it's like any other pregnancy from a medical perspective. A surrogacy pregnancy is also just like any other pregnancy, except you've got some extra people involved. The surrogate may show up at her doctor's appointment with her husband and two gay men in tow, or with her lesbian partner and a heterosexual couple, or whatever. But the physical process is the same as with any other pregnancy.

It's important that a surrogate's obstetrician be fully informed about the situation. An agency can help with this, but the responsibility lies with the surrogate to communicate what's going on—another reason surrogates need to be good communicators. Unfortunately, there are a few doctors who won't take these cases, as they philosophically do not approve of a woman carrying a baby for someone else. They just say no. Or they'll take the case, but they won't let anyone in the room except the surrogate. It's the doctor's decision who gets to be in the room, and that's the way it is. So if the parents want to accompany the surrogate for some or all of her appointments, the surrogate needs to choose an obstetrician who is open to that, and there are many who are. A doctor who is not comfortable with surrogacy is not the right doctor, no matter how knowledgeable or talented he or she may be. Be sure you establish this up front.

It's normal to be nervous during the pregnancy—especially if someone else is carrying your baby. But it's important to keep your expectations in check. Sometimes intended parents think their surrogate should be living in some sort of plastic bubble. I've had parents call me and they're apoplectic because the surrogate ate a candy bar. I just say, "Yup, she ate a candy bar. No problem." I mean, we do want surrogates to eat healthy food and take care of themselves, and we certainly don't want them smoking or drinking or guzzling caffeine, but a candy bar once in a while is really not a problem. But it's understandable that the parents want the surrogate safe and protected.

Sometimes I have to explain that nature has made the female body a perfect gestating machine. The body delivers whatever nutrients the baby needs, filtering out the junk. That said, we do want the surrogate to be living as healthy a lifestyle as she can and to be following all the doctor's directions.

Fact: If a pregnant woman is craving something, usually it's because there's something in it that she or the baby really needs. If she craves ice cream and pickles, her body may be telling her she's low on salt and sugar. So it's okay for her to eat the things she's craving as part of a healthy diet.

I've also had parents who read on Google that cat scratch fever can damage their baby, so they don't want their surrogate to have a cat. Other times they don't want a surrogate with a dog because they're worried the surrogate could be walking the dog and the dog could pull on the leash and she could fall over and land on her belly. All parents worry about all sorts of crazy stuff that's very unlikely to happen. But they only do that because they're nervous and they really want this to go well. Sometimes their fears just get the better of them. This is where, again, having an agency can help. They will provide a lot of support with a touch of education to get the parents through it, all the while validating how scary this process can be. After all, a surrogate is carrying the parents' most precious hopes and dreams and may be miles and miles away from them.

There can be legitimate disagreements, too. For instance, a surrogate might want to go hiking and camping at twenty weeks, and the parents may not be comfortable with that. If something like this happens, it's best to work with a third party (counselor, lawyer, agency) to mediate a solution. But remember, the only person who can officially tell a surrogate what to do or not do is a doctor. If the obstetrician says, "You're too far along to go camping and hiking," then she can't go. Otherwise, it's her decision. Typically, surrogates are very eager to please the intended parents and will follow their wishes as long as they are not unnecessarily restrictive or controlling.

Once in a while, I get calls from the surrogate asking me to intervene with the parents, instead of the other way around. The surrogate will say, "They call me every single night and ask what I had for dinner. Plus, they want to know about my bowel movements. Can you please tell them to calm down?" And this is fine. I would much rather a surrogate expresses her frustration or irritation to me than have her let loose with the parents. I actually tell our surrogates, "We can take as much frustration as you can dish out, so call us up and talk to us about it if you have to." But most surrogates don't. They take it all in stride, because they've been pregnant before. The only difference is they've got a few more people digging in their business this time. And they understand that intended parents' anxieties come from how much they already love and want their baby.

Higher Order Births (Twins, Triplets, etc.)

There is something very magical about twins, and many twin pregnancies work out wonderfully. However, it is important to note that higher order pregnancies (twins, triplets, and the like) are more complicated and higher risk. Twins have triple the normal perinatal (during the pregnancy) mortality rate, and triplets have six times the normal perinatal mortality rate. Twins are 50 percent more likely to be born prematurely, and with triplets that number goes up to 80 percent. Pregnant women are three times as likely to experience serious pregnancy-related consequences with twins and seven times as likely with triplets.

Chris and Sam were thrilled when their surrogate became pregnant with twins, and everything was going wonderfully in the pregnancy. Their surrogate's twenty-three-week appointment with the obstetrician couldn't have gone better, and she left the office with encouragement from her doctor to keep doing whatever she was doing. That night, though, things changed. Her water broke, and babies Kate and Alex were born—over four months early. Both babies weighed around two pounds. The odds of their survival were slim, and their health, if they survived, precarious. New dads Chris and Sam rushed to the hospital and spent the next 160 days camped out in the NICU, tube feeding their tiny precious babies the pumped breast milk that their surrogate delivered daily. With the love of their incredible daddies and the support of their surrogate, their families, and their nurses and doctors, Kate and Alex are now thriving toddlers. Not every story works out so well, but miracles abound in the world of assisted reproduction, and Kate and Alex are proof of that.

Planning for Potential Complications

Nobody wants to think about the things that can go wrong during pregnancy. However, especially in the case of third-party assisted reproduction, it's imperative that everyone involved be fully informed about the possibilities, with any and all potential complications discussed long before the embryo transfer takes place. That way a general plan of action can be agreed upon, well in advance, by all parties. Every contingency is explored, including the possibility of a therapeutic termination if there is something found to be wrong with the developing baby.

Legally, a surrogate cannot be forced to do anything with her body that she doesn't want to do. If she needs an abortion or the parents decide, for whatever reason, that they want her to have an abortion, but she decides she doesn't want to do that, then it's not going to happen. And nobody can force the issue. It's her body, and she can choose whether to have an abortion. This reality is another reason why my agency screens our surrogates as thoroughly as we do. We need to be certain a surrogate will carry out the parents' wishes—because it's their baby and their family, not hers.

Let me be perfectly clear here: nobody wants to have an abortion. It is not a callous decision on anyone's part. But sometimes a twelve-week ultrasound shows a fetus with no brain, or no kidneys, or some other major problem, and the baby is not going to make it—or if it does make it, the child may have a very poor quality of life. At that point, the parents must make a choice. Socially and emotionally, it's their choice. If the intended mother is carrying the baby, she and her partner will make all the decisions with the help of their obstetrician and usually also a high-risk specialist. With third-party ART, legally it's the surrogate's choice, but because a good agency will usually screen so thoroughly and have talked about it a lot already, they probably won't have any issues. The surrogate has already agreed to honor whatever the intended parents decide. Still, there will be many conversations supporting everyone through it. This is one of the reasons many people choose to work with an agency—when things go wrong, there is someone there to mediate.

Chris and Jan implanted two embryos, hoping for twins, and one of the embryos split. So their surrogate was pregnant with triplets. We had discussed the risks of transferring two embryos prior to embryo transfer, so everyone knew there was a chance this would happen. Still, when triplets were confirmed, the couple talked to numerous doctors to once again weigh the risks and make the best decision for themselves and their surrogate. In the end, the information they got confirmed the decision they'd made before the transfer: that in the event of triplets they would reduce to one, to the embryo that hadn't split, because that was the least risky option.

The surrogate had already told us that she would have a fetal reduction or therapeutic abortion if the parents asked for it. It was their decision and she was on board with it, but she was understandably still very upset. She was crying and she was mad at the world. The parents were emotional, too. It was awful, so I went to the procedure to support the surrogate and the parents.

At the ultrasound, because the high-risk specialist always looks at the fetuses first, the doctor could see some serious problems with the twins, even at that early stage—an issue called twin-to-twin transfusion that sometimes happens with identical twins where one twin grows too quickly and the other too slowly. The surrogate and the parents were comforted in the knowledge that the odds of those two babies surviving were very, very slim, and if the parents had chosen to stay with triplets, the other baby might also have been lost. But it was still tough on everyone. Decisions like that always are. Chris and Jan ended up welcoming one healthy baby into their lives, and they know they made the right choice for their family.

Of course, all parents potentially face this type of issue during pregnancy, regardless of who carries the baby or how it was conceived. No matter how great the science is, no matter how closely we monitor the pregnancy process, no matter how careful we are, things do sometimes go wrong. And this is the perfect time to rely on your support network to get you through the challenges in the assisted reproduction process. There are also support groups that you can join to get you through, and some really good books you can read. And of course this is a good time to enlist the help of a mental health professional.

You Get the Baby You're Meant to Have

As I mentioned earlier, I had a hard time getting pregnant. Natalie and I used several sperm donors before we had success. And I even had an early miscarriage. Without doubt, each failed effort was heartbreaking. But then we were blessed with Abby, and later, Jenna. Abby and Jenna are the two children that Natalie and I were meant to have. Never, not even once, have we questioned this fact. There are a lot of children we could've had, but these are the two we got, and they are what make us a family.

This is also my experience with assisted reproduction. There are occasional tragedies, babies are lost, and families are devastated by these losses. But then, later, they end up with the child or children they're meant to have. I learned this a long time ago with my own girls, and I've seen it over and over with the families I've helped to create. This is the knowledge that carries me through the tough times. The universe has a plan. If your journey is difficult, you will find your own way to cope. Assisted reproduction is a roller coaster, and it is really important that you have tools with which to cope with the ups and downs. Finding an online or in-person support group, journaling about your experience and feelings, and meeting with a mental health professional are just some of the things that can help. Find whatever inspires you to keep going. Honor your feelings, anxiety, grief, and sorrow. They are normal when things are challenging. These are the hardest miles in the marathon.

I have a Facebook page bookmarked on my computer that I go to every time I face a difficult situation. The page belongs to a family I worked with, a gay couple named John and Bill, who are two of the nicest people I've ever met. Like many gay couples, they decided to try for twins, a boy and a girl, using one embryo fertilized by each father. Everything went well until very late in the pregnancy, when we discovered that something was seriously wrong with the boy. John and Bill were devastated, the surrogate was devastated, and I was devastated, because we knew the boy twin was almost certainly not going to make it. On delivery day, both babies were born. The boy, Gabriel, lived for only a few hours. The girl, Olivia, was born healthy.

Two years later, John and Bill decided to try for a second child. They used a frozen embryo fertilized by Gabriel's genetic father and they had another baby, a beautiful little girl named Vivienne.

When the process goes awry, when there's an unexpected left turn and tragedy ensues, I go to Facebook and I look at Vivienne. Vivienne exists because Gabriel didn't make it. I know that John and Bill probably don't think about things this way, because that's not how parents think. They still mourn the loss of Gabriel. They've got a picture of him when he was born, and they consider him their guardian angel. They probably don't equate the birth of Vivienne to the loss of Gabriel. But from a distance, I do. When parents have had a tragedy and they're devastated, I go online and look at pictures of Vivienne playing soccer or playing the violin in one of her gorgeous dresses with a huge smile, and I know that things are going to work out. We're all shattered in the moment, but there is going to be a Vivienne for these parents, too.

Vivienne helps me to trust the universe; she inspires me. You too must find your inspiration. At these times, your partner, friends, family, and whatever else you believe in can help. With their help and support, you can find the strength and the willingness to move ahead.

I think John and Bill might be surprised to learn that Vivienne is my beacon of hope. Or maybe not. Maybe they feel the same way. When something goes wrong in their lives, maybe they look at her and think, "Yeah, but there she is." And maybe other people who know their story do the same. This is not to imply that the loss of Gabriel has some sort of silver lining. The loss of Gabriel is horrible and tragic. But now there is Vivienne. So when parents are faced with a similar situation, I can tell them from experience that everything will work out the way that it's meant to work out. And I almost always have them come back later and tell me I was right.

For every story where things go wrong, there are dozens of perfectly normal pregnancies and deliveries. I have written about some of the potential problems because I think it's important to present the most realistic view I can of the ART process, and the simple, sad truth is that occasionally things don't go the way we'd like. To ignore that possibility would not be ethical. But most of the time the hurdles encountered are relatively minor—delays, not disasters. And every year thousands of babies are born healthy and full term through ART, surrogacy, and egg and sperm donation. And hopefully you have been able to put together a trusted team of loved ones and experts to help get you through it all.

Birth

From a medical standpoint, ART deliveries are like all other deliveries. But they're also magical. There is something special about that extra layer of love that's in the room. So many people have come together to make this moment a reality, with so many delays and setbacks and maybe even tragedies, that when the moment finally arrives, it's extra special. It is the glorious finish line that may have eluded the intended parents for years.

In the case of surrogacy, the parents are invited into the delivery room, of course, though they don't always want to be there. It's the same as with a husband and wife, where the husband is invited but he might decide he'd rather wait outside. Plus, the surrogate's husband or partner might also be there. The exception to this is if the surrogate is having a C-section, a surgical procedure where one or more incisions are made through the abdomen and uterus to deliver the baby or babies. (Typically, C-sections are only performed when a traditional vaginal delivery would put the woman's or the baby's life or health at risk.) With a C-section it is up to the doctor how many people will be allowed in the delivery room. If the parents are not in the room, they will be right outside the door, allowed in the moment the baby is delivered.

Single mom Sharon attended the birth of her baby with her parents, sister, and best friend from college. Not to mention the surrogate's husband. As this was a normal, easy, single-baby vaginal delivery, the obstetrician allowed the whole party in the delivery room. Surrogate Tracy told me that the look on the family's faces as they saw the baby girl being born, the first and only grandchild in the family, will fuel her soul for the rest of her life.

Traditionally, the woman who just gave birth is tended to in the delivery room while the dad goes to the nursery, where they clean and measure the baby. And then everybody is reunited. The process is similar with surrogacy, except both parents go to the nursery with the baby while the surrogate gets tended to, and then they all reunite. Some parents choose to spend time with the baby in the delivery room after birth instead of going to the nursery right away. The key here is that the baby doesn't ever have to leave the parents' sight once it is born. Some parents choose to have the baby put instantly on their bare chest. This skin-to-skin care is a way to encourage bonding for both baby and parents.[1]

This is the parents' choice and a beautiful moment. And with surrogacy everything is discussed ahead of time and the hospital is prepared for the family's choices. If the baby is born full term, and without complication, it's likely the parents can take their child home the next day.

Usually the surrogate wants to have a picture with the new family, because that's what it's all about for her—creating a family. And the family wants that, too, of course. It's a special moment for all of them when they're together. It's bittersweet because the relationship will change at this point, but it's also joyful because everybody has been working toward this one special goal. This is the finish line in the long marathon they've been running together.

Fact: Cord blood (blood from the umbilical cord) is rich in stem cells and can be used to treat diseases that harm the blood and immune systems. If you plan to bank cord blood, you will need to contact the bank ahead of time and they will provide a kit to take with you to the hospital when you deliver. The doctor does the rest, taking the sample and submitting it to the bank.

When you hold your baby for the first time, it's incredible. Seeing this is the best part of the process for the surrogates, too. Surrogates love watching the people they've just helped diaper their baby backward, get peed on, and spill formula, learning and enjoying those first moments. This is the ultimate goal for surrogates. Like I've said many times, the surrogate isn't making a baby, she's making a family, and this is the payoff. Of course she cries. I don't think I've ever had a surrogate not cry. But she's not crying because she's giving up a baby; she's crying happy tears for the family she's helped create. These are tears of joy.

After delivery, the ongoing relationship between the surrogate and the parents is very personal and depends on the people involved. Most parents and surrogates do stay in contact to some degree, whether it's as Facebook friends, exchanging holiday and birthday cards, or just a normal friendship that develops over time. But the surrogate is not the mom. She never was the mom and she never will be the mom. Whether there are two dads, or a mom and a dad, or a single parent, the surrogate is the surrogate. No more, no less. She's the person who carried the baby and helped to make the family. And because she is screened properly before being approved as a surrogate, she understands this right from the start. Her intention was never to become the baby's mother.

Many surrogates are willing to pump breast milk for the newborn, and if that's something the parents want, the agency will help to facilitate it. Once the parents go home, the surrogate can continue to pump, freeze, and ship the breast milk for as long as it works well for both the surrogate and parents. Some parents don't want breast milk at all and will feed their baby with formula right from the start. Pumping is a big commitment on the part of the surrogate since it's hard to pump without an infant latching on, which is what causes milk to come in. Pumping also must happen round the clock, much as a nursing infant would do, in order to keep up the milk supply. So this is not for everyone. But when it works it's a lovely addition to the surrogacy process.

Birth is the finish line of this marathon called assisted reproduction. The people who have come together to bring a child into the world this way have endured a long and sometimes difficult journey, on purpose, with one goal in mind: fulfilling a wish. Creating a family. No matter which path is taken to get to this point, the baby's birth is the culmination of patience, persistence, commitment, collaboration, intention, and a whole lot of love.

CHAPTER SEVEN

Telling Your Story

FROM THE TIME you first think about creating your family, you are also creating your family story. And it's important to think about how you will tell that story to your child, your family, acquaintances, and even strangers.

It might help to know that you are not alone.

Fact: According to the 2010 US Census, *less than 25 percent* of American families are made up of a husband and wife who have a mutual biological child. And when it comes time for the 2020 census data to be compiled and released, I suspect that number may be even smaller.

Telling Your Child the Truth

I believe very strongly that you should tell your child the truth about how he or she came into the world. And the earlier you do this, the better. That way, there is no shame surrounding the topic and you weave your family's truth into the fabric of your child's life, making it an integral and beautiful part of who he or she is.

The key is to be honest and to keep it simple. I also suggest that you tell the story as often as you can. Do it the same way you talk to your infant all the time, even though the baby can't understand what you're saying. All they hear at that point is, "I love you and I'm doting on you." But when they do begin to understand language, one of the first things they'll hear is how much you wanted them.

Fact: From the moment babies are born they begin to take in information about who they are, and by the time they are toddlers they start to develop a sense of themselves. All the while, they are collecting and storing information and creating a gradually fleshed out narrative about themselves and the world around them.

You can tell your child that he or she began as a wish. That you wanted them so much you got help from other people to have them. That it takes a part from a man, a part from a woman, and then a place for the baby to grow, and sometimes we need to get some of those things from other people. Remind your child that a whole bunch of love and planning went into building your family. Then, as your child gets older, you can add age-appropriate language and more specific and accurate biological information. The key is to tell the story proudly, repeat it often, and add details as your child gets older and more able to understand.

This does not, however, mean that you need to share every detail of your child's conception and birth with everyone you encounter. You don't. But you do need to tell your child the truth right from the start. You need to let your child know that you really wanted a baby and you had to jump through all sorts of hoops to make it happen, so that's what you did and you're glad you did it. When the truth is embraced and celebrated, your child will feel wanted and special and loved.

When my oldest daughter, Abby, started kindergarten, there was an incident on the playground. This was in 2001, and she was the only kid in school with two mommies. We got a call from her teacher, who told us that some kids had circled around Abby, wanting to know about her dad. "You have to have a dad. Where is your dad? Who is your dad? What do you mean you don't have a dad? All kids have a dad." Apparently, Abby puffed out her chest and yelled proudly, "I don't have a dad. Everybody does not have a dad." The teacher said she thought Abby handled it just fine and there was nothing we needed to do or worry about. She just wanted to let us know. And that was the end of that. From then on, the kids understood our family makeup and accepted it—because the acceptance started with Abby.

The takeaway from this incident is that Abby stood up for herself because she knew her story and she loved it, so she felt empowered to defend it. What you make normal for your kids will be normal for your kids.

It's natural for children to look to their parents to understand why they look the way they do. Should you decide to build a family through third-party assisted reproduction, you need to consider what you'll tell your child about their genetic makeup. This is true for all types of families. So let me be absolutely, perfectly, 100 percent clear about this: *Making up stories and keeping secrets about your child's conception and birth is a very, very bad idea.*

To illustrate this point, I will share my own story. I was not raised with my biological father. Shortly after I was born, my mom met a wonderful man named Rod and they fell in love. They got married when I was an infant, and Rod, the only dad I've ever known, legally adopted me. Eighteen months later they had my sister, and we lived happily ever after as a family.

As I grew up, I knew all about my dad adopting me when I was really young, even the part where they took me to court and I said "yes" when the judge asked me if I'd like Rod to be my adopted dad. I don't actually remember any of it because I was too young, but my dad and mom told me the story hundreds of times and it became a part of who I am. I always knew my dad wasn't my biological father, but I never questioned his love for me or my love for him. He was my dad and he was an awesome dad. Period.

Unfortunately, my mom made up a story about my biological father. She told me that they were married and living in San Francisco, and when she was pregnant with me, she drove to LA to visit her parents. While she was there, my father was killed in a car accident in San Francisco. So that was the story I knew, and it was part of me just like the adoption story. But, as I came to find out, none of this second tale was true.

When I turned eighteen, my mom sat me down and told me the real story about my biological father, which is that they were not married, she got pregnant, and she decided that she wanted me and that she was okay being a single mom. And she told my biological father, "If you're not going to be fully in her life, then you're out of the picture." Then, after she had me, she met my dad, they got married, and he adopted me.

I was shocked—not by the fact that my mom wasn't married when she had me, but by the fact that she'd kept this from me all those years. I actually had a mini identity crisis because the story of my life was that my dear, loving father had died in a car accident while my mother was pregnant with me. So I can tell you from personal experience that finding out your real story when you're eighteen or twenty years old is not ideal. I know that my mom thought she was protecting me from a story she thought would be hard for me to accept or understand, but the truth is always the best way to go.

So, whatever else you do as a parent, don't lie to your child about his or her origins. Please, just don't do it. Intended parents sometimes tell me, "I want to tell my kids the truth, but I'll tell them when they're ten." No! Tell them before they ever know anything else so it's part of the fabric of who they are and they never have to have that "Really? Seriously?" moment later on. No child wants to be lied to or have secrets kept from them. Plus, lies and secrets nearly always come out anyway, so why not be truthful up front?

I'll never forget the dad who called me when his daughter turned seven because he felt it was the right time to tell her the story of her conception. I asked what he'd told her to date, and he said he had told her that her "mom" lived in America (they lived in Europe) and had stayed in the United States after she was born. Oops. That was going to be a hard one to undo. I understood where he was coming from in telling her that story; he thought that would be easier for her to understand than the truth: that she had no mommy and had been conceived through the help of an egg donor and surrogate. He thought he was doing the most loving and protective thing.

If you are worried that your child, your partner, or the world might not consider you to be a legitimate parent if you are not biologically related to your child, you shouldn't be. Love is what binds a family, not genetics. Regardless of whose genetic material you use, you and your partner are going to be full and equal parents. For instance, I have two wonderful daughters. I am biologically related to one but not the other. Yet I have never questioned my status as a parent with either. I don't ever think of one as mine and one as Natalie's. They're just our kids. And the same was true with my parents. I'm biologically related to my mom but not my dad. But that wasn't important to me. What mattered was that they both loved me. This will be true in your family as well. Genetics matter, but they are not what make a family. Love makes a family.

I have worked with parents who worry that when their child becomes a teenager he or she will resent being born through alternative methods. Rest assured that the teen years will be challenging, but that's something all parents deal with regardless of how their family was created. If you're two gay men, or you used an egg donor, or you're acutely uncool, or whatever, your teenager will use that as ammunition. If you're the slightest bit insecure about some aspect of your life, teenagers will figure it out and attack you with it. Because that's what they do. But that doesn't mean they don't love you. And research supports this: adolescents born through ART are just as healthy and well adjusted as other kids.[1]

I once worked with a woman who told me that she and her teenage daughter were sitting in the car on the way to the mall, stuck in traffic. The mom was driving and her daughter was in the passenger seat, and they were silent. And then the daughter started huffing and sighing, and the mom finally said, "What is it?" The daughter answered, "I just can't stand the way you breathe." So yeah, teenagers can be ridiculous. But that has nothing to do with their origin story.

If you tell your kids from the beginning who they are and where they came from, you will have built a foundation of confidence and trust. You let them know that there is nothing wrong with the way they came to be, and that it actually took more love than normal to make them. When this is their story, they know, in their hearts and souls, that there is nothing wrong with the way they and their family came to be.

Happily, things are different than when Abby started school, and people are more accepting. Mostly. You are still going to meet the occasional person who is uninformed and predisposed to judge you and your family and the way it was created. So be it. You can do your best to educate that person or you can sit quietly and ignore them. Either response is fine. But whatever you do, do not hide the truth from your child, because if you do that, you are tacitly agreeing with these ignorant individuals and their misguided beliefs.

Fact: According to the Williams Institute, between 2 million and 3.7 million children under the age of 18 have an LGBTQ parent.

Sharing Your Story Outside the Family

Telling people that you're expecting a baby is a very personal thing, regardless of how your baby was conceived and who is carrying your baby. In this respect, assisted reproduction is just like any other pregnancy. You might want to shout it from the mountaintops the moment you get a positive test, or you might prefer to wait for confirmation of a clinical pregnancy. Many people wait until the twenty-week ultrasound, when they are as sure as they can be that things are going well.

You should tell people about the pregnancy whenever you feel comfortable. Regardless of whether you tell others right away or wait until much later in the process, if something goes wrong, you're going to be devastated and you'll need support from the people who care about you. So you might want to tell the people you are closest to sooner rather than later. But if you prefer to wait, that's fine, too.

Of course, when you tell people you're expecting a baby, whether you are pregnant or a surrogate is helping you, you need to be prepared to answer a lot of questions. Some people will want to know the details, and you should be comfortable sharing that information if you've decided to share the news. Honesty is generally the best policy. If a surrogate is helping you, then say so. You can simply state, "We have this nice woman named Jane, and she's carrying our baby because we're not able to do that on our own."

Even well-meaning people will say ridiculous things and ask outrageous questions. For instance, after my second daughter was born my mother-in-law said, "Now you each have one." To which we said, "No, now we both have two. And you have two grandchildren or you have no grandchildren." She understood, and she's never mentioned it again. But still, she said it, and we had to respond to it.

Other ridiculous questions we've been asked more times than we care to count include: "Which of you is the real parent?" and, "Which of you is the mom, and which of you is the dad?" Anytime your family doesn't look the way a traditional family is expected to look, you can expect questions. When you use a third party to help you, whether a donor or a surrogate, some people will initially not understand.

Fact: Since 1978, eight million babies have been born through IVF.

Most of the time, people are not deliberately rude. Instead, they're curious, they're uninformed, and they don't know how to phrase their questions in a diplomatic way. Unfortunately, sometimes their curiosity goes too far and they ask about stuff that's really private.

If this sort of crazy-making Q&A worries you, I suggest that you and your partner (if you have one) plan a few stock answers in advance, such as, "We're both the real parent." Then, if you decide you want to occasionally elaborate and give more information, you can do so. But choosing to reveal information (especially about your child's genetic makeup) is your decision. You don't have to share that information just because someone asked. Your story belongs to you and your child, so you can share it or withhold it as you please. Just don't withhold it from your child.

Scotch and Todd are a couple who eventually transferred three embryos—two fertilized using one father's sperm, and one fertilized using the other father's sperm—after several unsuccessful single embryo transfer attempts. This time, all three embryos implanted, and they ended up with triplets. Happily, the babies were born healthy, and now they are the most adorable family you've ever seen. Scotch says, "Because our kids have always looked so different from one another, we constantly have to tell people they're triplets, after which they stare at our kids for a long moment and say, 'Are the girls twins?' To which we reply, 'No, they're triplets.'"

When people find out you're having your baby through surrogacy, they also might ask: "How do you know the surrogate is not going to just keep your baby?" In fact, it's almost certain that one of your family members, most likely your mom, will ask this question. The best option is to educate her; explain that the surrogate is carrying *your* baby and giving it back to you when it's born. You can also say that you're working with a reputable agency, that you've done your homework, that the surrogate has been fully screened, and that there are legal protections in place to protect your rights. Or you can just hand her a copy of this book. You'll be surprised how often the nervous nellies in your life become your staunchest allies and strongest supporters once they are informed and understand the process.

The Kids Are Definitely Alright

Should you choose to build a family through assisted reproduction, you may be wondering how your children will fare in life. There is a lot of research on this subject, and that research overwhelming supports the idea that kids born through assisted reproduction tend to do just fine. For instance, kids born to LGBTQ parents do as well (or better) on every measure of mental health and social adjustment.[2] Single parents also do a great job as parents.[3] And research shows that kids born through ART are healthy and well adjusted.[4] Moreover, the vast body of adoption[5] and ART literature[6] makes it crystal clear that openness and honesty lead to the healthiest outcomes.

I hope that knowing about all this research will help to reassure you about your choice to create your family through third-party assisted reproduction and help you know that being open and honest with your kids from the start will always be best.

Conclusion

LIKE RUNNING A MARATHON, building a family with assisted reproduction requires commitment, dedication, and endurance. The journey begins with a wish and then when you take your first step by walking into an agency, a law firm, or a medical practice. You meet the principals of the agency and learn about their process, and do your own research. If you decide to retain the agency, you are screened, contracts are signed, and you begin your search for a donor (if you need one). More contracts are signed, the agency matches you with a surrogate (if you need one), more contracts are signed, eggs are harvested and fertilized, embryos are tested and transferred. And you're only halfway there! You've still got nine more months of waiting before you hold your baby in your arms.

Fact: In third-party assisted reproduction the process from start to finish typically takes eighteen to twenty-four months—from starting the process to holding your baby in your arms.

For obvious reasons, building a family in this unique way brings out the best and the worst in people. It's normal to feel frustrated by the twists and turns that inevitably exist on the path. The legal contracts and paperwork may sometimes feel insurmountable. You might worry about the expense or resent the fact that you have to rely on a lot of other people to make such a deeply personal wish come true. But if you focus on the goal—creating the family that you have dreamed of—you'll find yourself doing whatever it takes to become a parent. And the wait will be worth it.

One pair of men among the first batch of intended parents through surrogacy was very anxious and hard to calm. Back then, third-party assisted reproduction existed in mostly uncharted waters, so the process wasn't always smooth and perfect. There was no template, and no experience to draw on. We were breaking ground every single day, knocking down barriers and battling with every ounce of energy we had because we believed in the endgame. Only a few doctors were willing to work with gay men, there were no laws protecting intended parents, and lots of people disagreed with what we were doing. In short, nothing was easy.

This couple had an absolute gem of a surrogate, but the process was bumpy and long. Their surrogacy journey was before there were systems in place, and they were understandably stressed and anxious throughout the process. With our encouragement, partnership, and support, they stuck with it and had a beautiful baby girl.

Sometimes parents are put through the wringer. Everything that could possibly go wrong does. They pick an egg donor, the retrieval is scheduled, but the donor gets her period the day before. We reschedule, but at the retrieval she only has a few eggs. We reschedule again, and this time there are ten eggs to fertilize. But when the doctor checks the five-day blasts, none of them look right. So we have to schedule another egg retrieval. Then, the embryo is transferred but it doesn't implant. Then the second try doesn't take. Then we transfer two embryos, hoping one will implant, but they both implant so now the intended parents have twins, which is not what they originally wanted, although they are thrilled. Then, at seven months, the surrogate has to go on bed rest, and she ends up delivering two months early. There are some harrowing days in the NICU since the babies were early and tiny, and their health and outcome are in question many times in the eight weeks they had to stay in the NICU. But the babies are healthy—they just need to grow and develop and pass through some developmental milestones, like breathing on their own and feeding well. Every time I see these parents or talk to them, they tell me how happy they are to be parents and how grateful they are to have the family they have.

People do this journey the way they do life in general, but magnified. Their strong points shine through, their anxieties take steroids. Assisted reproduction is like standing thigh-deep in water at the ocean's edge. If you resist the waves, you'll get knocked over. If you dive into the waves, you'll swim out the other side. It doesn't always go as planned, but much of the time what happens instead is better than the plan. How you choose to deal with the problems, both small and big, will determine your remembrance of the process.

Your Future Family Is Possible

Whatever your attitude toward the third-party assisted reproduction process, if you are patient, your family will happen. And the fact that you may or may not be genetically linked to your child will turn out to be inconsequential to you. The stranger who contributed to your child's genetic makeup is a part of your family's story, and a very important part, but you are your child's family. Third parties run the first part of your marathon with you, and sometimes for you; but then, when your baby is born, you take over. You'll definitely see things in your child that you will attribute (rightly or wrongly) to your donor, but you will also see yourself. Regardless of genetics, your child will in many ways be a reflection of you.

As you read this, you'll probably have a vision of who and what you want your child to be. You have an image in your mind. Well, that's not necessarily nor exactly what you're going to get. Studies show that personality is a mixture of nature and nurture. My daughters have the same sperm donor, but they're totally different. In some ways they're like the donor—both have his green eyes—in others they're like Natalie or me. But in all ways they're exactly who they're supposed to be.

Natalie and I met our sperm donor when Abby was six and Jenna was three. He was telling us about what he was like as a child, and he shared that when he was really young he would go to people's houses and come home with a bag of their trash, and then he'd create sculptures and machines out of it. Natalie and I just about fell out of our chairs, because Abby was notorious for grubbing through other people's wastebaskets and making sculptures and machines with what she found. She would go to somebody's house for a playdate and come home with a bag of aluminum foil and egg cartons. It was amazing to find out that our donor had done the same thing. Abby sure as heck didn't pick that up from Natalie or me. Neither of us is even remotely interested in touching other people's garbage. Who would think something like that was genetic?

Every parent I have ever worked with has stories like that. Kids are clearly a mix of their genes as well as the environment they grow up in. They do crazy things and parents have no idea where it came from. But it's mixed with personality traits that completely mirror one or both of the parents, regardless of biology. That's what makes each family unique and what makes raising kids so fun. They are who they are, and they will constantly surprise and amaze you. They begin as a wish, and that wish becomes reality. Maybe it's not always the reality you envisioned when you started your journey toward parenthood, but it's certain to be a reality that you wouldn't trade for any other.

Acknowledgments

CREATING YOUR FAMILY through assisted reproduction is a collaborative effort. It takes a village. The same can be said for my experience writing this book. There are so many people I want to thank. I am incredibly lucky and grateful to have such a vast and supportive village.

I want to start by thanking my incredible business partners, Stuart Bell, Erica Horton, and Teo Martinez, who always have my back and make me feel like a superstar. I also want to thank my dedicated staff at Growing Generations, who make it all look easy. I could not ask for a better team. Thank you also to all the doctors, lawyers, mental health providers, agencies, and other industry folks who lift this field up every day. It is an absolute pleasure to make this magic with you. I'd especially like to thank Dr. Mark Leondires for the beautiful foreword and for his medical expertise. And I absolutely want to thank my dear friend and reproductive attorney, Will Halm, who got me into this business to begin with when he casually asked me if I wanted to "help him help people have babies." Thank you for this amazing journey you set in motion.

Thank you from the bottom of my heart to all the parents who've trusted me to share their journeys to parenthood, especially the ones who have allowed me to tell their stories in this book. You are why I do what I do. I also want to thank the egg and sperm donors who have given of themselves so that someone else could become a parent. (I thank the sperm donor who helped me create my family every day in my mind!) And I want to thank the amazing and huge-hearted surrogates who I've had the pleasure of working with and who make it all possible. You are truly extraordinary.

I want to thank all the people who helped me write this book, from those who encouraged me to those who slogged through the editing, particularly my agents, Rick Richter and Rob Arnold at Aevitas Creative, who believed in the need for this book and never gave up; and Christine LeBlond, senior acquisitions editor at Red Wheel/Weiser, who saw this book's potential and tirelessly answered all my questions and helped turn my ideas into something people would want to read, allowing me to fulfill my dream of putting it all on paper. Thank you to my friend and attorney, Dan Mayeda, who is always there for me, and Scott Hamilton, who helped me find just the right words.

Last but certainly not least, I want to thank my loving family and friends. First, I want to thank my mom and dad, who showed me what truly unconditional love is and instilled a strong sense of family in me from the beginning. I am so grateful to Rabbi Denise Eger, who has been through every milestone with my family and provides a constant spiritual foundation for me and my family. I want to thank all of my friends who believe in me and are there for midnight pep talks, especially Diana Morgan, Susan Rosales, and Arleta Soares, who were on this journey with me every step of the way. I also want to thank my huge extended family of aunts, uncles, sister, brother-in-law, and cousins who buoy me always and show me what family means. I am truly blessed. And of course I want to thank Natalie, my amazing wife, best friend, and partner in all things, and my daughters, Abby and Jenna, who gave me the greatest gift in life: motherhood, the best thing I've ever experienced and the reason I want the same for anyone else who wants to be a parent and needs a little extra help.

Resources

Below is a list of resources to help you on your path to parenthood. I personally know every one of the companies, professionals, and organizations that I recommend below. If you are working with an agency, they will likely refer you to the professionals you will need to help you through your journey and the agency will put all the pieces together. I've listed many reputable agencies below in the Surrogacy, Egg, and Sperm Donation Agencies and Resources section.

Assembling Your Team

If you are planning to create your family through third-party assisted reproduction but you want to do so independently, please make sure that you include each of the following professionals on your team:

- A medical specialist, your reproductive endocrinologist —the doctor who will coordinate your IVF process.

- A reproductive attorney—a law practice dedicated to assisted reproductive law and family formation (parental rights) law, representing all types of clients including intended parent(s), surrogates, egg donors, embryo donors, and sperm donors (known as a full-service firm).

- A mental health professional specializing in fertility and ART.

- A fertility insurance expert—to help you obtain all of the different insurance policies that you will need.

You can start with the doctor, the lawyer, or the mental health professional, and they will be able to guide you to the other professionals and components that you need.

Medical Resources

ASRM Find a Health Professional:
www.reproductivefacts.org/resources/find-a-health-professional
A complete list by state of participating medical doctors and practices in fertility and assisted reproduction.

Fertility IQ: *www.fertilityiq.com*
Online community support and education and an extensive database of medical facilities with reviews.

Reproductive Endocrinologists

California Fertility Partners: *www.californiafertilitypartners.com*

Fertility Center of Las Vegas: *www.fertilitycenterlv.com*

Huntington Reproductive Center: *www.havingbabies.com*

Reproductive Medicine Associates Connecticut:
www.rmact.com

San Diego Fertility Center: *www.sdfertility.com*

Southern California Reproductive Center: *www.scrcivf.com*

Legal Resources

ASRM Find a Legal Professional:
www.reproductivefacts.org/resources/find-a-health-professional A complete list by state of participating legal providers in fertility and assisted reproduction.

International Fertility Law Group: *www.iflg.net*

International Reproductive Law Group: *www.irlawgroup.com*

The Law Firm of Meyers & O'Hara: *www.meyersohara.com*

The Law Offices of Amy Demma: *www.eggdonationtoday.com*

Reproductive Law Center: *www.rlcsd.com/index.html*

Steve Snyder, Esq.: *www.snyderlawfirm.com*

The Surrogacy Law Center: *www.surrogacy-lawyer.com/*

Vorzimer/Masserman Fertility and Family Law Center: *www.vmfirm.com*

Mental Health Resources

ASRM Find a Health Professional:
www.reproductivefacts.org/resources/find-a-health-professional A complete list by state of participating mental health providers in fertility and assisted reproduction.

Fertility Insurance Resources

Art Risk Financial and Insurance Solutions:
www.artrisksolutions.com

New Life Agency: *www.newlifeagency.com*
A full-service provider of assisted reproduction insurance.

General Fertility Resources

Below is a list of general fertility resources and support groups that can be very helpful during the ART process:

American Society for Reproductive Medicine (ASRM):
www.reproductivefacts.org

Multidisciplinary organization dedicated to the advancement of the science and practice of reproductive medicine. Full array of resources for people pursuing reproductive services including guidelines for surrogacy, egg and sperm donation, fertility practice statistics and success rates, and research. Also provides search engines for member doctors, attorneys, fertility practices, and mental health providers.

Fertility Road: *www.fertilityroad.com*
An online magazine for anyone looking to start a family. Parents share their experiences with international and domestic adoption, foster care, donor insemination, surrogacy, and parenting with an ex-partner.

Pregnantish: *www.pregnantish.com*
An online magazine and community dedicated to helping people dealing with infertility and fertility treatment.

Resolve: *www.resolve.org*
National fertility organization providing advocacy, education, community, and empowerment to all on the journey to family building.

Single Mothers by Choice: *www.singlemothersbychoice.org*
Provides peer support and information to women who are considering or have chosen single motherhood.

Surrogacy Agencies and Resources

All Things Surrogacy: *www.allthingssurrogacy.org*
Provides resources, education, and support for everyone in the surrogacy community.

A Perfect Match: *www.aperfectmatch.com*
A worldwide surrogacy and egg donor agency.

Center for Surrogate Parenting: *www.creatingfamilies.com*
A worldwide surrogacy agency.

Circle Surrogacy: *www.circlesurrogacy.com*
A worldwide surrogacy and egg donor agency.

Donor Concierge: *www.donorconcierge.com*
Conducts extensive searches of databases to help families
choose donors and surrogates.

Extraordinary Conceptions: *www.extraconceptions.com*
A worldwide surrogacy and egg donor agency.

Families Through Surrogacy: *www.familiesthrusurrogacy.com*
Provides worldwide conferences, seminars, and web resources
bringing together parents, surrogates, families, and experts.

Gifted Journeys: *www.giftedjourneys.com*
A worldwide surrogacy and egg donor agency.

Growing Generations: *www.growinggenerations.com*
A worldwide surrogacy and egg donor agency.

Reproductive Possibilities: *www.reproductivepossibilities.com* A
worldwide surrogacy matching agency.

Society for Ethics in Egg Donation and Surrogacy:
www.seedsethics.org/

Egg Donation Resources

A Perfect Match: *www.aperfectmatch.com*
A worldwide surrogacy and egg donor agency.

Beverly Hills Egg Donation: *www.bhed.com*
A worldwide egg donor agency.

Circle Surrogacy: *www.circlesurrogacy.com*
A worldwide surrogacy and egg donor agency.

Donor Concierge: *www.donorconcierge.com*
Conducts extensive searches of databases to help families choose donors and surrogates.

Extraordinary Conceptions: *www.extraconceptions.com*
A worldwide surrogacy and egg donor agency.

Fairfax EggBank: *www.fairfaxeggbank.com*
One of the largest egg banks, with locations around the country.

Gifted Journeys: *www.giftedjourneys.com*
A worldwide surrogacy and egg donor agency.

Growing Generations: *www.growinggenerations.com*
A worldwide surrogacy and egg donor agency.

Parents Via Egg Donation (PVED): *www.pved.org*
Educates, supports, and empowers families and individuals at any stage of the process who choose to use egg donation to build a family.

Sperm Donation Resources

California Cryobank: *www.cryobank.com*
Frozen donor sperm and egg bank providing family building services to intended parents around the world. Also provides cord blood banking.

Fairfax Cryobank: *www.fairfaxcryobank.com*
Sperm bank providing sperm to families worldwide.

Financial Resources

Baby Quest: *www.babyquestfoundation.org*
Provides financial help for infertility treatment.

Cade Foundation: *www.cadefoundation.org*

Provides information and financial assistance to families overcoming infertility.

Nest Egg Foundation, Inc.: *www.nesteggfoundation.org*
Provides grants of up to $10K for IVF services.

New Life Fertility Finance: *www.newlifefertilityfinance.com*
Provides financing for fertility treatments and insurance.

LGBTQ Resources

Children of Lesbians and Gays Everywhere (COLAGE): *www.colage.org*
Support and empowerment for people with LGBTQ parents or caregivers.

Family Equality Council: *www.familyequality.org*
National organization dedicated to advocacy, resources, education, and support for LGBTQ families, including family-building resources. Includes extensive database of research and parenting support.

Gayparent.com: *www.gayparentmag.com*
Longest running nationally distributed publication dedicated to LGBTQ parents and parents-to-be.

Gay Parents to Be: *www.gayparentstobe.com*
An informational resource and link to LGBTQ family building resources

Men Having Babies: *www.menhavingbabies.org*
Provides resources and education for gay men pursuing biological fatherhood.

Pop Luck Club: *www.popluckclub.org*
Long-standing resource and support group for gay dads and dads-to-be.

Endnotes

CHAPTER ONE

1 Kimberley Lipschus, "How a Skeleton Grows New Skin: Transformation for the Reproductive Client," *Gestalt Journal of Australia and New Zealand* 13, no. 2 (May 2017): 91.

CHAPTER TWO

1 This is best discussed in Maggie Kirkman, "Saviours and Satyrs: Ambivalence in Narrative Meanings of Sperm Provision," *Culture, Health & Sexuality*, 6, no. 4 (July 2004): 319–334.

2 Patricia P. Mahlstedt, Kathleen LaBounty, and William Thomas Kennedy, "The Views of Adult Offspring of Sperm Donation: Essential Feedback for the Development of Ethical Guidelines Within the Practice of Assisted Reproductive Technology in the United States," *Fertility and Sterility* 93, no. 7 (May 2010): 2236–2246; Vasanti Jadva, Tabitha Freeman, Wendy Kramer, and Susan Golombok, "The Experiences of Adolescents and Adults Conceived by Sperm Donation: Comparisons by Age of Disclosure and Family Type," *Human Reproduction* 24, no. 8 (August 2009): 1909–1919.

CHAPTER THREE

1 Alex Lopata, "History of the Egg in Embryology," *Journal of Mammalian Ova Research* 26, no. 1 (April 2009): 2–9.

2 Susan Caruso Klock, Andrea Mechanick Braverman, and Deidra Taylor Rausch, "Predicting Anonymous Egg Donor Satisfaction: A Preliminary Study," *Journal of Women's Health* 7, no. 2 (March 1998): 229–237; and Z. Brew, K.

Bergman, R.-J. Green, and K. Katuzny, "Motivations and Personality Characteristics of Egg Donors Who Help Gay Men Become Parents via Gestational Surrogacy," (unpublished research manuscript, In Press. Presented as October 20, 2014). Egg donors working with gestational surrogacy agencies: Motivations and personality traits. Research Poster, American Society for Reproductive Medicine (ASRM) Convention, Honolulu, HI.

CHAPTER FOUR

1   The Countway Library Repository Archive assembled by the Francis A. Countway Library at Harvard Medical School.

2   Eyal Fruchter, Ronit Beck-Fruchter, Ariel Hourvitz, Mark Weiser, Shira Goldberg, Daphna Fenchel, and Liat Lerner-Geva, "Health and Functioning of Adolescents Conceived by Assisted Reproductive Technology," *Fertility and Sterility* 107, no. 3 (March 2017): 774–780.

CHAPTER FIVE

1   Nancy Wieland Troy, "The Time of First Holding of the Infant and Maternal Self-Esteem Related to Feelings of Maternal Attachment," *Women & Health* 22, no. 3 (1995): 59–72; Mario Mikulincer and Victor Florian, "Maternal-Fetal Bonding, Coping Strategies, and Mental Health During Pregnancy—The Contribution of Attachment Style," *Journal of Social and Clinical Psychology* 18, no. 3 (September 1999): 255–276; Anna Hjelmstedt, Ann-Marie Widström, and Aila Collins, "Psychological Correlates of Prenatal Attachment in Women Who Conceived After In Vitro Fertilization and Women Who Conceived Naturally," *Birth* 33, no. 4 (November 2006): 303–310.

2   A. Anderson, K. Bergman, R.-J. Green, and S. Pardo, "Motivations and Personality Characteristics of Gestational Surrogates Who Help Gay Men Become Parents," (unpublished research manuscript, In Press. Presented as August 9, 2014). Motivations, decision making, and MMPI-2 scores

of surrogates willing to help gay men become parents. Research poster, American Psychological Association (APA) Convention, Washington, DC.

CHAPTER SIX

1 Réjean Tessier, Marta Cristo, Stella Velez, Marta Girón, Zita Figueroa de Calume, Juan G. Ruiz-Paláez, Yves Charpak, Nathalie Charpak, "Kangaroo Mother Care and the Bonding Hypothesis," *Pediatrics* 102, no. 2 (August 1998): e17.

CHAPTER SEVEN

1 Susan Golombok, Elena Ilioi, Lucy Blake, Gabriela Roman, and Vasanti Jadva, "A Longitudinal Study of Families Formed Through Reproductive Donation: Parent-Adolescent Relationships and Adolescent Adjustment at Age 14," *Developmental Psychology* 53, no. 10 (October 2017): 1966–1977.

2 Susan Golombok, Lucy Blake, Jenna Slutsky, Elizabeth Raffanello, Gabriela D. Roman, and Anke Ehrhardt, "Parenting and the Adjustment of Children Born to Gay Fathers Through Surrogacy," *Child Development* 89, no. 4 (January 2017): 1223–1233; R.-J. Green, R.J. Rubio, K. Bergman, and K.E. Katuzny, "Gay Fathers by Surrogacy: Prejudice, Parenting, and Well-Being of Female and Male Children," (paper presentation August 7, 2015, American Psychological Association (APA) Convention, Toronto, Ontario).

3 Thomas Deleire and Ariel Kalil, "Good Things Come in Threes: Single-Parent Multigenerational Family Structure and Adolescent Adjustment," *Demography* 39, no. 2 (May 2002): 393–413.

4 Viveca Söderström-Anttila, Ulla-Britt Wennerholm, Anne Loft, Anja Pinborg, Kristlina Aittomäki, Liv Bente Romundstad, and Christina Bergh, "Surrogacy: Outcomes for Surrogate Mothers, Children and the Resulting

Families—a Systematic Review," *Human Reproduction Update* 22, no. 2 (March–April 2016): 260–276; H. Bos and F. van Balen, "Children of the New Reproductive Technologies: Social and Genetic Parenthood," *Patient Education and Counseling* 81, no. 3 (December 2010): 429–435.

5   Betsy Keefer Smalley and Jayne E. Schooler, *Telling the Truth to Your Adopted or Foster Child: Making Sense of the Past* (Santa Barbara, CA: Praeger, 2015).

6   Elena Ilioi, Lucy Blake, Vasanti Jadva, Gabriela Roman, and Susan Golombok, "The Role of Age Disclosure of Biological Origins in the Psychological Wellbeing of Adolescents Conceived by Reproductive Donation: A Longitudinal Study from Age 1 to 14," *Journal of Child Psychology and Psychiatry* 58, no. 3 (December 2016): 315–324.

Index

placenta, 50
pre-birth judgment, 70
pregnancy, 89–100
    care of surrogate during, 91–94
    chemical pregnancy, 89–91
    clinical pregnancy, 89–91, 111
    complications, planning for potential,
      95–98
    complications, prior to 6-week mark,
      89
    concerns of parents about surrogate,
      92–94
    early miscarriage, 89–91, 98
    getting the baby you're meant to have,
      98–100
    higher order, 94–95
    hormone treatments after embryo
      transfer, 89–91, 111
    therapeutic termination of (abortion),
      94–95
preimplantation testing, 54–56, 60
premature birth, 94–95
progesterone injections, 91
prostate, 14
psychological evaluation of surrogate, 72

R

relatives
    as donor egg donor, 42
    screening, 75
    as surrogates, 75, 78–79
reproductive attorney, 6–7, 123
reproductive endocrinologist (medical
    specialist)
    cost of, 9–10
    in egg retrieval process, 40
    qualifications of, 4–6
    resources, 124
    in screening surrogate, 72
    in sperm donation, 18
residence requirements for surrogates,
    70, 71
Rock, John, 48

S

Schleiden, Matthias Jakob, 31
Schwann, Theodor, 31
screening
    egg donors, 35–38, 43
    embryo, 54–56
    genetic, 54–56
    goal of, 75
    parents, 75–77
    relatives as surrogates, 75
    rescreening repeat surrogates, 74

by sperm banks, 21–22
sperm donors, 21–28
surrogates, 69–75
truth in, 76–77
scrotum, 16
semen, 14
seminal vesicle, 14
sex of baby determined by timing of
    insemination, urban legend of, 23
sex selection, 56–57
sexually transmitted diseases (STDs), 16,
    21, 32, 51
speculum, 87
sperm, 13–28
    anonymous donors, 43–46
    in conception through heterosexual
      intercourse, 15
    correcting issues, 16–17
    description of, 14–15
    ducts, blockage of, 16, 17
    freezing, 20, 22, 32
    of HIV-positive men, 17–18
    hormonal issues, 16
    infertility, 16–17
    partner being allergic to, 51
    period of male fertility and, 14
    potential problems, 15–18
    process of generating and delivering,
      14
    science of, 13–15
    screening process, 21–28
    testing, 16
    varicocele, 16
sperm banks, 18, 20–22, 23
    anonymous donors, 23
    location of, 20
    process of sperm donation, 20–21
    screening process, 21–22, 35
sperm donation, 18–21. *see also* sperm
    banks
    anonymous donors, 23–24
    characteristics of donor, 20
    choosing donor, 23–25
    compensation for, 34–35
    disclosure of donor, 25–26
    female couples, issues in, 27
    history of, 19–20
    home inseminations, 22
    intelligence testing, 21
    male couples, issues in, 26–28
    process of, 20–21
    resources, 129
    screening of donors, 21–28
sperm extractor, 21
sperm washing, 17–18

About the Author

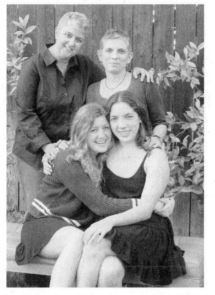

Kim Bergman (top right, with her family)

Kim Bergman, PhD is a licensed psychologist and co-owner and senior partner of Growing Generations, one of the oldest and largest surrogacy and egg donor agencies in the world. Based in Los Angeles, she is a well-respected expert on assisted reproduction, serves on the corporate board of the American Society for Reproductive Medicine, and is an emeritus board member for the Family Equality Council. Visit her at *www.growinggenerations.com.*

To Our Readers

Conari Press, an imprint of Red Wheel/Weiser, publishes books on topics ranging from spirituality, personal growth, and relationships to women's issues, parenting, and social issues. Our mission is to publish quality books that will make a difference in people's lives—how we feel about ourselves and how we relate to one another. We value integrity, compassion, and receptivity, both in the books we publish and in the way we do business.

Our readers are our most important resource, and we appreciate your input, suggestions, and ideas about what you would like to see published.

Visit our website at *www.redwheelweiser.com* to learn about our upcoming books and free downloads, and be sure to go to *www.redwheelweiser.com/newsletter* to sign up for newsletters and exclusive offers.

You can also contact us at *info@rwwbooks.com.*

Conari Press
an imprint of Red Wheel/Weiser, LLC
65 Parker Street, Suite 7
Newburyport, MA 01950
www.redwheelweiser.com